CATCHING FIRE

CATCHING FIRE

Women's Health Activism in Ireland and the Global
Movement for Reproductive Justice

Beth Sundstrom and Cara Delay

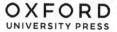

OXFORD
UNIVERSITY PRESS

OXFORD
UNIVERSITY PRESS

Oxford University Press is a department of the University of Oxford. It furthers
the University's objective of excellence in research, scholarship, and education
by publishing worldwide. Oxford is a registered trade mark of Oxford University
Press in the UK and certain other countries.

Published in the United States of America by Oxford University Press
198 Madison Avenue, New York, NY 10016, United States of America.

CIP data is on file at the Library of Congress

ISBN 978–0–19–762510–1 (paperback)
ISBN 978–0–19–774394–2 (hardback)

DOI: 10.1093/oso/9780197743942.001.0001

This material is not intended to be, and should not be considered, a substitute for medical or
other professional advice. Treatment for the conditions described in this material is highly
dependent on the individual circumstances. And, while this material is designed to offer
accurate information with respect to the subject matter covered and to be current as of the
time it was written, research and knowledge about medical and health issues is constantly
evolving and dose schedules for medications are being revised continually, with new side
effects recognized and accounted for regularly. Readers must therefore always check the
product information and clinical procedures with the most up-to-date published product
information and data sheets provided by the manufacturers and the most recent codes of
conduct and safety regulation. The publisher and the authors make no representations or
warranties to readers, express or implied, as to the accuracy or completeness of this material.
Without limiting the foregoing, the publisher and the authors make no representations or
warranties as to the accuracy or efficacy of the drug dosages mentioned in the material. The
authors and the publisher do not accept, and expressly disclaim, any responsibility for any
liability, loss, or risk that may be claimed or incurred as a consequence of the use and/or
application of any of the contents of this material.

Paperback printed by Marquis Book Printing, Canada
Hardback printed by Bridgeport National Bindery, Inc., United States of America

For reproductive justice advocates past, present, and future—including the activists who shared their stories and inspired this book.

CONTENTS

Acknowledgments   *ix*

Introduction   1

1. Cervical Cancer Prevention   20

2. Contraception   46

3. Abortion   74

4. Pregnancy   103

5. Childbirth   129

6. Obstetric Violence: Symphysiotomies and
   Hysterectomies   153

Conclusion   183

Notes   *191*
Resources and Further Information   *233*
Index   *243*

ACKNOWLEDGMENTS

Writing this book has been a highlight of our careers and collaborations, and we are grateful to all who have supported us. We are particularly thankful for our Fulbright US Scholar Research Grant Awards in Ireland, which allowed us to complete research for this project, and for the communities we were fortunate to join at University College Dublin and University College Cork. We would also like to thank our colleagues at the College of Charleston. The School of Humanities and Social Sciences, the Departments of History and Communication, the Women's and Gender Studies program, and especially, the Women's Health Research Team (WHRT) have provided encouragement and assistance. Our work with faculty and students on the WHRT has inspired and energized us throughout this process. We are most appreciative of our collaborations with WHRT members, past and present, and particularly Ryan Murphy, Mackenzie Pelletier, Brooke Harris, Kaitlyn Victoria, Logan Elkins, Kate Davis, and Madeline Ashby, who helped us conduct research related to this manuscript.

We are indebted to our community of scholars, women's health activists, and organizational partners in the United States and abroad, who make our research not only possible but also rewarding. We thank our colleagues at the Medical University of South Carolina, the University of South Carolina, Clemson University, Brown University, the Women's Rights and Empowerment Network, the South Carolina Coalition for Healthy Families, Fact Forward, the South Carolina Cancer Alliance, the St. Jude Children's Research Hospital HPV Cancer Prevention Program, Power to Decide, Free the Pill, and Ibis Reproductive Health, among others, for collaborating in our essential research on women's health.

The editorial team at Oxford University Press has been a joy to work with. Sarah Humphreville has been supportive and enthusiastic at every step of this process. We also extend our gratitude to *Éire-Ireland*/The Irish-American Cultural Institute and Emerald Publishing for permission to reprint portions of previously published articles.

We owe the success of our research to the activists and advocates who participated in our interviews. We are grateful for your generosity in sharing your time, experiences, and voices. Your stories and voices, which we hope we have done justice to here, are invaluable and need to be heard.

Our friends and families, especially Paris, Bryan, Millie, and Byrdie, have shown us such patience, encouragement, and generosity of spirit. Thank you for the time and space to write, and thank you for listening.

Introduction

In the aftermath of the successful 2018 vote to repeal Ireland's divisive anti-abortion Eighth Amendment to the Constitution (1983)[1] and pave the way for legal abortion, author Maeve Higgins captured the sentiments of the feminist activist community when she wrote in *The New York Times*, "There's this feeling I get . . . in Ireland, particularly among women, and I wish you could feel it, too, because it's extraordinary. It's something like electricity but really a more ancient source of power, like fire, and the thing about fire, of course, is that it's catching."[2] Higgins's likening of women's health activism to a natural source of power taps into traditions of feminine influence in Irish culture and also conjoins the past and present, nodding to the essential historical precedents of recent "electric" activism in Ireland. Her categorization of fire as a contagious force references the extraordinary potency and diffusion of women's health activist movements in Ireland, which have indeed been "catching," helping not only to overturn abortion restrictions but also to legalize same-sex marriage (2015); move toward woman-centered healthcare, such as by reforming CervicalCheck and enacting the Coroners (Amendment) Act 2019 requiring an official investigation into all maternal deaths; and, currently, lead the call for further inquiries into the Magdalene laundries and Mother and Baby Homes.[3]

By shedding light on the essential work of activists, including ordinary people utilizing digital activism, and examining activist

Catching Fire. Beth Sundstrom and Cara Delay, Oxford University Press. © Oxford University Press 2023.
DOI: 10.1093/oso/9780197743942.003.0001

methods and messages, this book investigates how and why women's health movements in Ireland "caught fire." Over the past few decades, organizations and activists have mobilized to protest how Irish women have been harmed, and continue to be harmed, by a misogynistic healthcare system steeped in a damaging neoliberal, postcolonial, and Catholic ethos.[4] *Catching Fire* focuses on attempts by Irish healthcare reformers, organizations, social media contributors, and campaigners to address the wrongs of the past and improve Irish women's[5] access to essential healthcare services. Linking Irish developments to global movements, it also places recent activist campaigns in an essential, yet often overlooked, historical context. Irish activists and advocates employed a strategy of truth-telling, making women's narratives and embodied experiences the central focus of their movements, and engaged with a variety of media outlets to spread their message and enact change. In particular, activists utilized technology to their benefit, contributing to the growing field of feminist digital activism. Moreover, their approach of empowering ordinary women to tell their own stories through ethical communication has resulted in widespread compassion and solidarity. This strategy, we argue, has personalized reproductive justice and established the Republic of Ireland as a model for future global activist movements. In fact, the successful example of *In Her Shoes*, a 2018 campaign on Twitter and Facebook that helped convince Irish voters to overturn restrictive abortion legislation, has been mimicked in places like Gibraltar, where activists also have sought to reform restrictive abortion laws.[6]

APPROACHES AND METHODS

In their essential essay exploring the possibilities of transitional justice in Ireland, Katherine O'Donnell, Maeve O'Rourke, and James M. Smith ask, "What is it that Ireland still needs to learn about its treatment of women, children, and others marginalized by poverty, sexism, racism, ageism, and ableism both in the past and in the present?"[7] As we argue in this book, how and why women's bodies and reproductive experiences were at the heart of this oppressive "treatment" of women and children remains understudied. A plethora of important recent research has shed light on the institutions that comprised what James Smith calls Ireland's "architecture of containment" and Caelinn Hogan refers to as "the shame-industrial complex."[8] Still, most works continue to explore the legal, political, and religious contexts of these institutions; what happened to the infants and children who entered or were born in institutions; the circumstances that led to women's incarceration in Magdalene laundries and Mother and Baby Homes; or who was/is "responsible" for these institutions and the harm they created.

While these are all essential areas of study, the real-world embodied experiences of women and all people who can become pregnant both inside and outside of these institutions have been largely left behind. And scholars' focus on institutions, while welcome and important, has sometimes obscured how Irish women were metaphorically incarcerated in other spaces of Irish society, including homes, hospitals, and healthcare providers' offices. In this book, while we reference women's health within the institutions that comprised the "shame-industrial complex," we also broaden the conversation to underscore the importance of misogyny in women's health. We analyze a series of representative examples and case studies that demonstrate most clearly the work of activists: the cervical cancer prevention crisis, contraception, abortion, pregnancy, childbirth, forced hysterectomies, and symphysiotomy. We build on the work of Claire Bracken and Cara Delay, who argue that "the island's history of institutionalization in Magdalen laundries, asylums, and Mother and Baby Homes should also be read alongside the realities of inadequate healthcare for women and their oppressions by and through the medical establishment."[9] This is a significant issue when studying a country that placed multiple meanings, and enacted violence, on women's real-world bodies. As Clara Fischer writes, "the moral purity at stake in the project of Irish identity formation was essentially a sexual purity enacted and problematized through women's bodies."[10] It is to women's embodied realities and healthcare experiences, then, that we must turn our attention.

Recently, Irish Studies scholars and activists working on the Magdalene laundries and Mother and Baby Homes have pointed out the need to feature the voices and narratives of survivors and, where possible, victims—those "who have been too frequently ignored."[11] "In Irish efforts to address historical abuse across a range of contexts," writes James Gallen, "power remains out of the hands of victim-survivors and of those traditionally marginalized in society."[12] In this book, we attempt to feature the voices of those affected by healthcare harms; the activists and activist organizations whose work has been, and is still, essential to changing the culture of women's healthcare in Ireland; and the ordinary Irish people who became changemakers through digital activism.

We have also responded to the call by scholars that research on digital feminist activism should address intersectionality in order to understand social movements.[13] Through the lens of digital intersectional communication theory, we examine the ways that social media advocacy and intersectionality impact truth-telling in women's health activism.[14] We adopt an intersectional framework and analysis, recognizing the extent to which scholarship on reproduction and healthcare in Ireland has been limited by a focus on white, middle-class, cis-gendered, and straight individuals. Such an approach does not illuminate real-world experiences or realities in Ireland today. In 2019, for example, migrant and ethnic minority women comprised 40% of maternal deaths in Ireland.[15] An activist we interviewed problematized the reality that some parts of the 2018 movement to

repeal anti-abortion statutes were "overwhelmingly white," pointing out that migrant and disabled women, along with those living
in Direct Provision, "where you know parents can't make the most
basic decision about how to parent their children, and you know,
kind of living in this isolation and degradation being institutionalized," are particularly burdened under the existing system. Another
activist wrote of the Repeal movement, "For the most part, we didn't
hear from the messier edges of the campaign, from the places where
multiple oppressions occur to squeeze people of their rights. There
was no place in this exceptionally respectable campaign for the sex
worker, the woman with a psychosocial disability, women of colour,
migrant women, Traveller women, trans men. They were sacrificed
for the greater good."[16]

Since Repeal, the healthcare realities of marginalized groups
have further come to light, especially as the system of Direct
Provision, which houses asylum-seekers, has been criticized and
rethought. Katie Mishler categorizes Direct Provision as an heir, or
even a continuance, of the "shame-industrial complex." "Migrants
and women of color in the asylum system," she writes, "continue
to be subjected to the same biopolitical control as so-called 'fallen
women' in the last century."[17] Similarly, the work of the advocacy
group Migrants and Ethnic-minorities for Reproductive Justice
(MERJ) has underscored how the Irish state persists in subjugating
migrants and people of color. MERJ was born in 2017 in order "to
create a platform for the often hidden faces and voices of migrants
and ethnic minorities in Ireland that were all but missing from Irish
feminism."[18] Furthermore, as Fiona de Londras and others have
pointed out, the post-Repeal Health (Regulation of Termination of
Pregnancy) Act (2018) harms transgender and nonbinary people
who may need abortion "as a result of the government's refusal to
add 'pregnant person' to the statutory descriptor of those accessing
care under the law."[19]

Also essential to an intersectional framework is a recognition and exploration of the ways in which women's healthcare activism has long built from, and intertwined with, other forms of activism. Bridget Keown writes, for example, "The theoretical foundations that gave rise to the gay-rights movement and subsequent marriage referendum of 2015 are the same that led to the movement to repeal the Eighth . . . Both focused on the harm—physical, emotional, spiritual, and psychological—done by prevalent heteronormative notions of identity, citizenship, autonomy, and health."[20] Steph Hanlon, activist in Carlow, Ireland, explains that abortion-rights activist organizations did not, and do not, focus solely on abortion: "We were long-time activists who campaigned during the water charges movement, the marriage referendum, are now active in Extinction Rebellion . . . we originated in 2017 due to the struggle for abortion; however, during that time we've lobbied for other issues i.e., housing, childcare, trans rights, etc."[21]

To best explore the complexities of health discrimination and activism in Ireland, *Catching Fire* offers a mixed-methods approach. It features archival research, document analysis, interviews with activists, and participant observation. Participant observation included more than twenty hours of informal meetings with experts and activists in Ireland. Qualitative observations involved open-ended discussions and activities documented in unstructured field notes.[22] The document analysis portion of the study included an examination of published documentation and archival records, as well as traditional and social media. Archival research was conducted at the National Archives, Dublin; the National Library, Dublin; the *An Bord Altranais* (Nursing and Midwifery Board) Archive, Dublin; and the Boole Library, University College, Cork. Archival materials include documents from the Irish women's movement spanning the 1970s to the 1990s, the records of *An Bord Altranais*, and government documents such as directives and surveys from the Health Department.

In examining these archival sources, we recognize their limitations as documents created primarily by white, cis-gendered individuals representing the viewpoints of organizations or the government. In the Irish archives, this shortcoming is particularly evident. We therefore draw here on recent scholarship that has created an imperative for doing more than simply reading so-called "traditional" documents "against the grain."[23] We attempt to focus on not only whose stories the archives tell but also "how stories are told" and what stories are often left out.[24]

To access some of the historical actors whom traditional archives overlook, we also examined published sources, including feminist journals, newsletters, newspapers, government reports, and autobiographies/memoirs. We collected publicly accessible documents (websites, press releases, reports, tweets, Facebook posts, YouTube videos, etc.) from twenty women's organizations. Finally, we searched for news and key figures on Twitter and Facebook to provide additional evidence. Therefore, this research highlights both traditional and social media, which have been essential to women's health activism. Materializing from a history of silence and stigma, women's voices have been amplified by technology and social media. Activists and advocacy organizations have been instrumental in raising awareness of, and support for, monumental social and cultural change, including through digital story-telling and multimedia projects, such as the documentary *Picking up the Threads* by filmmaker Anne-Marie Greene and the short film *Silent Killer: A Timeline of the DEATH of Savita Halappanavar* by Laura Fitzpatrick. In recent years, visual digital culture and art has emerged as "a key site through which to track and consider forms of activist story-telling beyond the narrative threads of the written word."[25]

Interviews were conducted with health activists in Ireland in 2018 and 2019. Purposive sampling was used to recruit interview participants based on predetermined criteria. In addition, we asked participants to refer other activists, offering a "snowball" sampling approach to maximize requisite variety. Interviews were robust in both length and depth, lasting over an hour at in-person locations convenient for participants or via Skype. Interviews were digitally recorded and transcribed verbatim. All data were combined into the evidentiary database. Some of the activists we interviewed shared concerns about being identified and requested anonymity. In order to fully respect these wishes and maintain consistency, we will quote all participants in our research without identifying them by name. The reproductive justice framework and a constant comparative method provided a rigorous, inductive approach to data analysis to identify patterns and themes across the data.

Throughout, we employed feminist research methods, which are committed to intersectional analyses that acknowledge participant and researcher standpoints.[26] Feminist inquiry explores the lived experiences of women as creators of knowledge and makes the impact of gender visible where it was hidden.[27] The overall aim of feminist research is to support social justice and redress inequities that impact the lives of women and other oppressed groups.[28] This book builds on Donna Haraway's call to disrupt the nature/culture duality to move beyond essentialism in order to understand how technology may be used to support women.[29] Following feminist science studies, our analysis demonstrates social construction of knowledge and explores technoscience outside of hegemonic process to reimagine gender, sex, and nature.[30] In a global context, we addressed power and intersections of difference by engaging in dialogue with multiple forms of difference.[31] We employed feminist interviewing to value the voices and lived experiences of women in Ireland. As a result, feminist interviewing methods address the power imbalance in the researcher-researched relationship by focusing on relationships.[32] As women's health activists ourselves, we validated relationships with our participants through self-disclosure, "woman-to-woman" talk, and reciprocated nurturing, promoting true dialogue by empowering participants to serve as co-researchers rather than subjects of our research.[33]

GLOBAL RIGHTS AND REPRODUCTIVE JUSTICE

The conceptual framework of *Catching Fire* is reproductive justice. Reproductive justice is itself grounded in a global human rights context. In 1994, the International Conference on Population and Development (ICPD) declared that women's rights are human rights—and that these rights depend on each person's ability to determine *if, when, and how* to have children.[34] Furthermore, the conference established that women's health is inextricably intertwined with women's empowerment and gender equality more broadly. Around the same time, a group of American Black women met in Chicago to create the reproductive justice movement, which centers the needs of women of color and other marginalized people who had been largely overlooked by traditional women's rights movements in the twentieth century.[35] SisterSong, the largest national multiethnic reproductive justice collective in the United States, defines reproductive justice as "the human right to maintain personal bodily autonomy, have children, not have children, and parent the children we have in safe and sustainable communities."[36]

Reproductive justice is based on human rights and requires bodily autonomy for all people. Reproductive justice goes further, arguing that individual human rights are indelibly linked to larger social, historical, cultural, and structural issues that must not be ignored. Reproductive health includes fertility management, childbirth, and parenting, which are fundamental human rights.[37] As a result, reproductive justice advocates for a social safety net provided by the government to ensure access to the basic necessities parents need to raise their children in a safe and healthy environment. Kimala Price writes that reproductive health and rights are connected to other social justice issues, including education, economic justice, poverty, housing, immigration policy, environmental justice, drug policies, prisoners' rights, and violence.[38] Violence includes institutional and state-sponsored violence that impacts women's reproductive health, such as policies that reflect neoliberalism, colonialism, white supremacy, criminalization, and capitalism. A reproductive justice approach aims to understand and dismantle the systems of social inequality that shape, oppress, and restrict reproductive rights and health access.

Both a human rights framework and reproductive justice are essential to understanding the Irish context. Since at least the 1990s, health activist organizations and individuals have consistently challenged national laws and policies by holding the state accountable to global human rights policies. As a member state of the European Convention on Human Rights, for example, Ireland has agreed to protect its citizens' "right to life." Health activists have argued that this applies to Ireland in the case of maternal healthcare, which, as scholar and activist Jo Murphy-Lawless's work has elucidated, has consistently fallen short in protecting and preserving maternal lives.[39] Tanya Saroj Bakhru argues that in response to crises such as the 2012 death of Savita Halappanavar, the Irish Family Planning Association (IFPA) "responded with a call to action based on human rights discourse," underscoring "the discrepancies in Irish law, service provision and international human rights covenants to which Ireland was a signatory."[40] By referencing a human rights framework, Irish activists have provided a clear legal rationale for their proposed reforms and also, significantly, have linked Ireland with global and transnational movements to guarantee the rights of individuals. Murphy-Lawless, however, points to the need for a more comprehensive reproductive justice analysis: "There is an acute need to analyze the resulting structural inequalities that the neoliberal state has both fostered and denied in order to see more clearly the myriad ways in which they impact women's lives."[41]

In Ireland and beyond, activists and organizations addressing women's health have sought to combine a human rights perspective with a more encompassing reproductive justice framework. Several interviewees we spoke to articulated the need for Irish health activists to privilege reproductive justice. One talked about a "kind of totality about how we understand reproductive injustice and maternal death and maternal morbidity and access to contraception and home use of the abortion pill, and you know I thought all of this was part of this same story." According to another activist, "I also think the perception of motherhood, there's a whole debate that's going to have to happen around fertility and infertility and working mothers, women who don't have children and work, there's a lot of issues there that we haven't seen in Irish society, that we could see come out in the debate."

Although Ireland appears to be a more homogeneous society than the United States and thus may not obviously lend itself to an analysis of the intersections of race, gender, and class that reproductive justice demands, recent examples involving the Traveller community, migrants, and people of color in Ireland point to its changing demographics and the resulting need for a more nuanced investigation. In addition to the 2012 Savita Halapannavar case, when Indian-born Halapannavar died after being refused a therapeutic abortion in a Galway hospital, the 2010 examples of pregnant Nigerian migrant Bimbo Onanuga, who died at Dublin's Maternity Hospital, as well as "Applicant C," a Lithuanian migrant who sought an abortion in Ireland, testify to the unique challenges faced by migrant women in Ireland.[42] Furthermore, examinations of how Ireland's historical "others," including not only religious minorities or historical migrant groups (e.g., post-WWII Hungarians) but also the Traveller community, its indigenous ethnic minority group, have demonstrated that the supposed historical homogeneity of Irish society is more construction than reality.[43] Investigations of Traveller women's reproductive experiences in particular have exposed a system that marks these women as different and "pathological."[44] The reproductive justice movement's emphasis on the intersections of gender, class, and race/ethnicity therefore is directly relevant to the Irish case.

Furthermore, in the Irish context, reproductive justice also offers a conceptual lens to understand the island's unique colonial and postcolonial past and present. Clara Fischer has written about "the stubborn persistence of the denial of reproductive rights to women in Ireland over the decades by arguing that deep-seated, affective attachments formed part of processes of postcolonial nation-building that relied on shame and the construction of the Irish nation as a particular, gendered place."[45] Ireland's women were long subjugated under the British colonial system and were defined after Irish independence as bearers of the new postcolonial nation. As a result, their bodies were contained and controlled in variety of contexts, including through the religiously informed and medicalized reproductive healthcare system. As is common in colonial and postcolonial contexts, traditional women's health practitioners in Ireland, known as handywomen, were targeted as dirty and "uncivilized" by colonial authorities. After independence, male religious, political, and medical leaders sought to continue the imperial "civilizing mission" and thus demonstrate that the new Ireland was worthy of self-rule.[46] A new focus on combating infant mortality and ensuring that Irish women acted as good mothers resulted in government-sponsored maternity and child welfare schemes that served almost 60,000 Irish women by the mid-1930s.[47] Concomitantly, professionally trained nurses and physicians became the designated experts on women's reproductive health, and throughout the next few decades, a modern biomedical paradigm overtook women's healthcare.[48]

Here, again, the Irish context was unique in the influence that the Catholic Church held over physicians.[49] In the late 1960s, Irish women composed letters to journalist Monica McEnroy of the magazine *Women's Way* about the obstacles they faced in regulating their fertility. One woman directly pointed out the links between the Irish medical profession and the Catholic Church, writing:

> I am thirty-eight. I have five lovely children. The eldest is eight and I have just lost another baby before its time. I have high blood pressure for the past two years. I asked my doctor could I not try the Pill as I want to try and look after the children. The worry of another miscarriage is always hanging over me, but he told me I would have to wait until they got word from Rome.[50]

Ireland's history of colonial domination requires a more in-depth analysis of ethnicity, religion, and otherness as they were, and are, mapped on women's reproductive bodies. Reproductive justice also applies to the Irish case when we consider that throughout much of the twentieth century, while married women were urged and coerced into having children, others—notably unmarried women who were incarcerated in Mother and Baby Homes and other punitive institutions—were denied "the right to *have* children."[51]

TRUTH-TELLING

Irish Studies scholars in recent years have explored the concept of transitional justice as a means of working through the harms of the country's violent institutional past. Although most commonly used in societies emerging from war or conflict, transitional justice has been applied more widely as a way to process and account for numerous historical harms and traumas, including, for example, in relation to Canada's troubling history of Indian Residential Schools.[52] In Ireland, transitional justice is being discussed as a potential approach in dealing with the history of the Mother and Baby Homes and Magdalene laundries.[53] While there is also a case to be made for categorizing hospitals as institutions that may fall under the purview of transitional justice, we find one particular element of the concept most useful in the Irish case: truth-telling. An activist we interviewed stated:

> I think truth-telling is an important aspect of reproductive justice because in international human rights law, one of the key human rights guarantee is nonrepetition, and I don't think you can guarantee nonrepetition if you don't know what you did. If you don't investigate the patterns of abuse that we were complicit in the past you can't guarantee something similar won't happen in the future.

In 2007, the United Nations described a "right to truth" for individuals, societies, and nations. Over the last half century, truth-telling in the form of truth and reconciliation commissions has been recognized as a central feature of postwar transition to enact justice and reparation.[54] Beyond the context of war and conflict, truth-telling offers a mechanism to document and condemn violations of human rights, which may or may not include judicial action.[55] According to Hala Bassel, truth-telling among the victims of enforced sterilizations in Peru served as a nonviolent method of historical justice that protected victims' right to the truth as a form of resistance and created the possibility of reparation.[56] Margaret Urban Walker argues that truth-telling by victims of injustice is a kind of reparation itself, though it is unlikely to be sufficient reparation.[57]

Although many scholars advocate for truth-telling as a form of healing for victims, Karen Brounéus argues that women who had participated in reconciliation tribunals in Rwanda experienced traumatization, ill health, isolation, and insecurity.[58] Similarly, James Gallen problematizes transitional justice as potentially patriarchal, writing, "Further criticism has suggested that transitional-justice practice retains a significantly genderblind approach, with the result that women are typically disadvantaged and deprioritized in the provision of testimony, accountability, prosecution strategies, and access to effective remedies and redress."[59]

Truth-telling requires an analysis of gendered contexts; therefore, truth-telling and reproductive justice go hand-in-hand. In most cases, truth-telling in response to violations of human rights is initiated by the state. However, Alison Crosby and M. Brinton Lykes investigated truth-telling introduced by civil society, which emphasized accountability by listening to women's voices, avoiding reifying or essentializing women's experiences, and affirming local women's meaning making.[60] It is this approach, which mirrors a reproductive justice framework, that can make truth-telling transformative. According to Gilmore, social media has democratized truth-telling, allowing new, credible speakers to emerge as power shifts.[61] There is a robust literature examining feminist digital activism related to intimate partner violence and rape culture.[62] One analysis of truth-telling in the #MeToo movement revealed "there was so much pain, carried over a lifetime, exacerbated by silencing, that poured into the public square."

Although not without its limits and problems, social media offers a platform to co-create health and illness narratives and share everyday lived experiences.[63] Kaitlynn Mendes, Jessica Ringrose, and Jessalynn Keller highlight the challenges and potential of digital feminist activism:

While being vehicles for incivility, misogyny, and abuse, digital platforms such as blogs, Twitter, and Tumblr simultaneously offer women a platform where they can communicate, form communities of support, engage in consciousness-raising, organize direct action, disrupt the male gaze, and collectively call out and challenge injustice and misogyny through discursive, cultural, and political activism.[64]

Online narratives enable individuals to see themselves in the stories of others, creating emotional and intellectual engagement.[65] In Ireland, social media has also provided an anonymous, decentralized platform, which created new opportunities for marginalized groups, such as Traveller, refugee, and asylum-seeking women, who may not have always been welcomed by mainstream movements, to engage in truth-telling.[66] As a result, truth-telling is particularly relevant to an analysis of reproductive justice and women's health in Ireland.

Catching Fire begins with an analysis in chapter 1 of the cervical cancer prevention scandals of the early 2000s. In 2015, Ireland saw a misinformation campaign about the human papillomavirus (HPV) vaccine that led to a sharp decline in Irish vaccination levels; just three years later, Ireland's CervicalCheck screening program came under scrutiny once it was revealed that it gave hundreds of women incorrect negative screening results, leading to several preventable deaths from cancer. However, women and public health advocates publicized and problematized these scandals, forcing a government response and demonstrating the power of truth-telling and ethical communication. They exposed systemic and endemic problems involved in women's healthcare in Ireland, including overinflating the authority of male doctors and the medical establishment's history of ignoring women's experiences and voices.

Chapter 2 moves to an analysis of contraception, arguing that access to birth control is one of the most essential issues facing people in Ireland today. Following the lead of activists and social media contributors, this chapter places contraception in conversation with other healthcare issues, notably abortion. It explores how and why those who have advocated for abortion rights in recent years also have prioritized access to contraception by adopting a reproductive justice framework. By dispelling harmful myths, confronting contraceptive ignorance and opposition, and sharing everyday embodied realities, activists and advocates ultimately helped convince the government to budget for free contraception, which was implemented in January 2023 for women and people with a uterus aged 17 to 26.

The analysis of abortion in chapter 3 highlights the importance of the Repeal campaign, which in 2018 helped lead to a successful vote overturing the anti-abortion Eighth Amendment to the Irish Constitution. In late 2018, the Health (Regulation of Pregnancy) Act legalized abortion up to twelve weeks in a pregnancy. The chapter analyzes both the methods and content of the Repeal movement, demonstrating its global meanings and links as well as how and why it resonated with so many Irish people. It also interrogates the efficacy of social media activism, asking what voices such campaigns featured—and what voices they sometimes obscured. Moving beyond legality to engage with reproductive justice, chapter 3 also underscores the importance of abortion access, which has remained limited since the 2018 Act and especially during the COVID-19 pandemic.

Chapter 4 turns to an examination of pregnancy, deconstructing issues of identity and power by explicating how medicalization has impacted the embodied experience of pregnancy in Ireland. Through a study of the National Maternity Strategy and current maternity practices, this chapter explores how calls for woman-centered care intersect with practices of midwifery and the biomedical obstetric paradigm. An analysis of the *In Our Shoes—COVID Pregnancy* social media campaign, which shared anonymous narratives from women impacted by COVID-19 restrictions in Ireland, highlights the current context of debates on pregnancy rights and activism. The COVID-19 pandemic magnified existing health systems issues and disrupted access to maternal health services, revealing how medicalization of women's bodies and the institutionalization of maternity services continue to regulate women's reproductive lives and result in systematic repression during labor and childbirth. Uncovering gender inequity in government policies during a time of crisis reveals the need for systemic change to ensure every women's human right to high-quality, respectful maternity care in all circumstances.

Chapter 5 explores the historical, social, and cultural impact of the medicalization and institutionalization of childbirth in Ireland. An analysis of the campaign for the Coroners (Amendment) Act 2019 led by the Elephant Collective reveals how feminist praxis successfully demanded mandatory inquests for maternal deaths. This chapter also examines the diverse ways that hospital births in Ireland undermine women's bodily experiences by privileging medical authority. It also reveals how the normalcy of hospital birth is supported by media, physicians, prenatal classes, and women's fears and desires for a safe birth. Finally, this chapter highlights the continued need for truth-telling to center women's lived experiences in order to disrupt the nature/technology dualism.

The book ends with an analysis of obstetric violence. Chapter 6 interrogates two case studies: the forced hysterectomy scandal at Our Lady of Lourdes Hospital during the 1990s and the symphysiotomy scandal that became public in the early 2000s. In the second half of the twentieth century, thousands of Irish women endured these harmful procedures at the hands of physicians empowered to abuse women's bodies. This chapter examines these incidents as examples of obstetric violence. These practices testify to the pervasiveness of religious, national, and biomedical power in Ireland, past and present. The chapter argues that in order to achieve reproductive justice in Ireland, we must confront obstetric violence, following the lead of survivors who have spoken out and told truths about their embodied realities and the harms they have suffered in Ireland's medicalized reproductive healthcare system.

CONCLUSION

Catching Fire, while focused on the Irish context in recent years, also brings comparative and historical insight to the topic of women's health activism. It places Ireland within a global context—particularly meaningful given the island's history of emigration and its active diaspora, as well as the attention that scholars have given to the healthcare needs of migrants and asylum-seekers in Ireland today. In particular, developing a human rights culture through grassroots organizing and truth-telling offers a model for US activists because "few people in the United States have opportunities to observe how the UN works or to learn about human rights in the terms internationally recognized outside the United States (i.e., a broader set of rights well beyond civil and political rights, including socioeconomic, cultural, and developmental rights)."[67] This book features the understudied roles of women's health activists who have challenged high-tech myth systems to redefine women's health and reproduction, making them central concerns in Irish society and government. This insight contributes to the disruption of the nature/culture dualism and highlights the possibilities of empowerment through technology in women's health. The Irish case offers important insight into understandings of gender, science, and technology in the global movement for women's autonomy. Furthermore, at a critical turning point for reproductive justice, Ireland's activist successes provide insight for pursuing global gender equality in the shadow of the COVID-19 pandemic.

Cervical Cancer Prevention

Human papillomavirus (HPV) is ubiquitous, and most people will be infected during their lifetime. Persistent infection can lead to six HPV-related cancers in men and women, including cervical cancer. Recent research suggests that widespread HPV vaccination and cervical screening could eliminate cervical cancer globally by the end of the twenty-first century. The Republic of Ireland, however, has faced significant challenges to widespread HPV vaccination and cervical screening in recent years resulting from the CervicalCheck cancer scandal and the HPV vaccination misinformation campaign. Applying a reproductive justice lens to Ireland's cervical cancer prevention crisis reveals the importance of truth-telling and empowering women to make decisions about their own bodies through a women-first approach to healthcare. By raising women's voices, advocates in recent years have engaged in story-telling about health, illness, and the body to confront, challenge, and change Ireland's healthcare system.

From 2015 to 2018, scandals surrounding HPV and cervical cancer screening in Ireland revealed serious deficiencies in the nation's healthcare system. In 2015, a misinformation campaign about the HPV vaccine resulted in a sharp decline in Irish vaccination levels, and in 2018, Ireland's CervicalCheck screening program was revealed to be flawed, providing hundreds of women with incorrect

Catching Fire. Beth Sundstrom and Cara Delay, Oxford University Press. © Oxford University Press 2023.
DOI: 10.1093/oso/9780197743942.003.0002

negative screening results and leading to several preventable cancer deaths. In the 2018 Scally Report,[1] a scoping inquiry into Ireland's CervicalCheck screening program, key informants pointed to the significant gendered failings of the Irish healthcare system, noting:

- "Why does it always happen to women?"
- "I think there is a history of looking at women's health services as being secondary."
- "Women and women's rights are not taken seriously."
- "Paternalism is alive and well." .

The Scally Report identified the need for expert and committed attention to women's issues within the healthcare system.

Through an analysis of two scandals, the CervicalCheck screening program and the HPV vaccination misinformation campaign, this chapter investigates the cervical cancer prevention crisis in Ireland through the lens of reproductive justice. HPV vaccination and cervical screening are health behaviors that illuminate the intersection of oppressions based on race/ethnicity, socioeconomic position, ability, age, gender, sexual orientation, and immigration status.[2] These categories are best analyzed through reproductive justice, which underscores intersectional oppressions in women's healthcare and advocates for truth-telling as resistance. Indeed, this chapter is one of the first studies to apply a reproductive justice approach to cervical cancer prevention, including HPV vaccination.

Both the CervicalCheck screening program and the misinformation campaign about HPV vaccination were rooted in unethical communication by the state and nongovernmental actors. Unethical communication is ingrained in hegemonic, paternalistic sociopolitical practices that mirror narratives of oppression based on gender, ethnicity, and nationality.[3] During the cervical cancer screening crisis, as a legal expert explained to us, "a number of op-eds in papers suggested that these [activist] women alone were going to bring down the CervicalCheck system and were going to destroy healthcare for other women." This provides clear evidence of unethical communication. In contrast, ethical communication is "socially oriented, empathically situated, and responsive to others."[4] In the midst of Ireland's cervical cancer prevention crisis, women and public health advocates confronted and resisted unethical communication through digital intersectional communication by engaging in story-telling and truth-telling about health, illness, and the body to confront, challenge, and change Ireland's healthcare system. Jennifer Vardeman and Amanda Sebesta propose a digital intersectional communication theory in which social media advocacy and intersectionality are connected, arguing that "the sociopolitical climate today simultaneously and equally demands transparency and reflexivity."[5] These scholars advocate for normative intersectional communication in socially mediated spaces to address the solidarity-discord identity paradox that emerges in social-mediated social justice advocacy campaigns.[6] By privileging the voices of activists and experts, we argue in this chapter that the ways women and public health advocates confronted the cervical cancer prevention crisis in Ireland may be understood as a triumph of ethical communication—primarily truth-telling and digital intersectional communication—over the failure of unethical communication. We contend that ethical communication is also an essential element of reproductive justice, although thus far it has not been studied explicitly as such. Reproductive justice demands that activists move beyond legal and political contexts to address social justice and community realities.[7]

CERVICALCHECK CANCER SCANDAL

Each year in Ireland, more than 6,500 women receive surgical treatment for pre-cancer of the cervix, about 300 women are diagnosed with cervical cancer, and almost 90 women die from cervical cancer.[8] Among women 25 to 39 years of age, cervical cancer is the second most common cause of death from cancer.[9] Almost all cases of cervical cancer are caused by HPV. Recent research suggests that widespread HPV vaccination and cervical screening could eliminate cervical cancer globally by the end of the twenty-first century.[10] In 2019, the World Health Organization (WHO) ramped up work to eliminate cervical cancer worldwide through a comprehensive approach to cervical cancer control and prevention, including increasing HPV vaccination and appropriate screening and treatment.[11]

In Ireland, CervicalCheck offers free cervical screening (formerly smear test) to women aged 25 to 60. The CervicalCheck cancer scandal first appeared in 2018, when it was revealed that more than 200 Irish women received false-negative screening test results and were not informed of the error. Some of these women subsequently became ill from cervical cancer and then sued Ireland's publicly funded health system, the Health Service Executive (HSE). One of these women was Vicky Phelan, who refused to sign a confidentiality clause as part of her settlement, thereby illuminating the failures of CervicalCheck, which included widespread nondisclosure of standard audits. According to the Scally Report,[12] over one million Irish women were screened between 2008 and 2015, with 1,067 cases of cervical cancer reported. Among those 1,067 cases, 300 required further review, and 204 women were found to have received incorrect results from before they were diagnosed with cancer. Although letters were sent to their healthcare providers, only 43 of the 204 women (or one in five) were informed about the results of the audit. Ultimately, the CervicalCheck cancer scandal revealed that a significant number of women could have been diagnosed earlier and avoided terminal disease or death.

HPV VACCINATION MISINFORMATION CAMPAIGN

Human papillomavirus is a common sexually transmitted infection (STI), and most people will be infected with a form of HPV during their lifetime. The body typically clears HPV on its own; however, when the virus persists, it can cause changes to cells that lead to cancer over time. According to the HSE, HPV causes 406 cancers in men and women every year in Ireland. A vaccine to prevent HPV infection has been licensed since 2006. According to Kate Simms and colleagues[13] 124 countries and territories include HPV vaccines in their national immunization programs. A school-based HPV vaccination program for girls 12 to 13 years of age was introduced in Ireland in 2010. The vaccine currently used in Ireland is Gardasil 9, which prevents approximately 90% of HPV-related cancers.[14] Over 270 million people have been vaccinated with Gardasil globally, including more than 260,000 people in Ireland. The Global Advisory Committee on Vaccine Safety considers HPV vaccines to be extremely safe.[15]

Despite the safety and effectiveness of the HPV vaccine, vaccine communication crises can result in vaccine hesitancy and low uptake. The WHO named vaccine hesitancy, which is the reluctance or refusal to vaccinate despite vaccine availability, one of the ten threats to global health in 2019.[16] In 2015, a misinformation campaign targeting HPV vaccination appeared in Ireland. The anti-vaccination campaign targeted parents and gained widespread coverage on social media, as well as local and national media. Designed to undermine trust in vaccines, the campaign publicized unevidenced and false testimonials of side effects, health problems, and injuries allegedly caused by the HPV vaccine.

Initially in Ireland, national rates of vaccination plummeted from approximately 87% to less than 40% of girls. However, a timely response brought the national average back up to approximately 75%

in less than five years. According to the WHO, this vaccine safety communication crisis was successfully addressed through coordination and engagement between key stakeholders, including health departments, immunization programs, influential public leaders, and the media.[17] This chapter identifies the ways that activists, in particular, contributed to this successful coalition through truth-telling.

REPRODUCTIVE JUSTICE

Reproductive justice requires bodily autonomy for all people and is grounded in human rights. According to Zakiya Luna:

> The work of organizing to create a human rights culture not only asks the government to create the conditions of human thriving but also pushes the public to understand themselves as deserving of these conditions *and* as having a role in maintaining human rights through respecting each other's human rights.[18]

This process is evident in Ireland's grassroots organizing and truth-telling to address women's health scandals. For example, the hepatitis C scandal emerged after pregnant women were administered contaminated anti-D immune globulin, manufactured by the Blood Transfusion Services Board (BTSB), to prevent RhD isoimmunization in RhD-negative mothers. The advocacy group Positive Action was formed to support women impacted by this failure of the healthcare system. One of the women infected with hepatitis C, Brigid McCole, brought her case to court to reveal the truth. McCole's truth-telling spurred the state to take action, publicly admitting liability and establishing a compensation tribunal in the late 1990's.[19] The hepatitis C scandal built a foundation for women's truth-telling and advocacy to demand redress from the state.

The cervical cancer prevention crisis provides clear evidence for the relevance of reproductive justice in contemporary Ireland. According to an interview we conducted with an Irish legal expert, these scandals reveal systemic issues:

> There are questions there about consent, about women's entitlement to knowledge about their own bodies, how women are spoken to when their reproductive function or sexual function is in question. There are questions about the gender dynamics that can take place between powerful and predominately male doctors and their female patients. There are questions about shame and stigma.

A reproductive justice approach aims to understand and dismantle the systems of social inequality that shape, oppress, and restrict women's health and reproductive rights.

We argue that the cervical cancer prevention crisis in the 2010s was mitigated by health activists applying reproductive justice to the Irish context. Reproductive justice acknowledges the complicated intersections of gender, race/ethnicity, socioeconomic position, immigration status, ability, sexual orientation, and age as sources of reproductive oppression based on systems of social inequality, including sexism, racism, classism, xenophobia, ableism, heterosexism, and ageism. This framework contextualizes the biological, economic, social, and political systems that shape women's access to and decision-making about cervical cancer prevention, including HPV vaccination, screening, and treatment.

Scholars also have called for reproductive justice research to better understand health disparities in cervical cancer prevention.[20] To date, however, most global research has failed to apply a reproductive justice approach to increase women's agency and empowerment in preventing STIs and cervical cancer, including HPV vaccination.[21]

Marginalized populations, such as uninsured and underinsured women, immigrants, and people of color are at increased risk for HPV infection and HPV-related cancers.[22] Research also suggests that women negotiate, and sometimes resist, cervical cancer screening. For example, a recent qualitative study found that Traveller women did not attend cervical screening because they viewed this preventive intervention as embarrassing and unimportant.[23] Therefore, we cannot underestimate the importance of ethical communication that provides a complete understanding of the risks and benefits of screening and overcomes medical control of women's bodies.[24] Effectively countering anti-vaccination movements requires communication that moves beyond essentializing women to their reproductive function and reconceptualizes normative, "natural" processes by countering the false duality of natural and technological related to vaccination, screening, and treatment.[25] An analysis of the cervical cancer prevention crisis uncovers historical, religious, and cultural contexts for reproductive justice and women's health in Ireland. This intersectional analysis improves understandings of health inequities, particularly among marginalized women, such as Traveller, refugee, and asylum-seeking women.

TRUTH-TELLING

Truth-telling in response to violations of human rights may be introduced by civil society to avoid essentializing women's experiences and affirm women's meaning-making.[26] In this way, truth-telling grounded in reproductive justice was transformative in the Irish context. When Vicky Phelan refused to sign a confidentiality clause, refusing to be silenced, she empowered women's voices and stories. When other women shared their experiences with cervical cancer on social media, they controlled their stories and demanded transparency and accountability. Scholars argue that social media has democratized truth-telling, providing an opportunity for new speakers to emerge as power shifts.[27]

This chapter investigates Ireland's cervical cancer prevention crisis in two parts, the CervicalCheck cancer scandal and the HPV vaccination misinformation campaign. We examine how the CervicalCheck scandal inspired women to confront a legacy of shame and silence around women's bodies and health, and how truth-telling empowered women to challenge systems of inequality. Our analysis of the HPV vaccination misinformation campaign shows how the HPV Vaccination Alliance, a group of more than thirty-five Irish organizations, charities, and public institutions that joined together in 2017, successfully countered HPV vaccine hesitancy by advocating for ethical communication, including truth-telling, in order to protect and advance the position of individuals in vulnerable situations. These crises are contextualized by social, economic, and environmental concepts, including gender, sexual orientation, race/ethnicity, socioeconomic position, immigration status, age, and ability.

CERVICALCHECK CANCER SCANDAL

In the mid-nineteenth century, doctors noticed that cervical cancer was rare among Catholic nuns, while being fairly common among other women. Although this observation would eventually lead to the first vaccine for cancer, it also stigmatized cervical cancer by linking it to sexual activity: "Prostitutes had a relatively high risk of contracting the disease, married women in town had a moderate risk, and the celibate nuns (with the unfortunate, presumably rare, exceptions) were spared. This epidemiological profile strongly suggested that a sexually transmitted agent played an important role in the development of cervical cancer."[29] Stigmatizing women's sexuality and shaming women for negative health outcomes emerged as a central theme in the 2018 Scally Report, in which Dr. Scally described "one of the most disturbing accounts" of a disclosure meeting in which the close relatives of a deceased woman were told that "nuns don't get cervical cancer."[30]

According to one of our interview participants, an expert on women's health in Ireland:

> My own take on it is that the same thing wouldn't have happened if it were men's health we were talking about, the way a lot of those women were spoken to by consultants and medical professionals was very gendered and it seemed to wrap up a lot of negative issues and ideas around women's sexuality, it was a medical issue that seemed to have a moral tone to it which it shouldn't have.

The healthcare system, government, and media perpetuated this stigma and shame by attempting to silence the women impacted by the scandal. Clara Fischer's politics of shame contends that "gendered shame may form a disciplining device operating through structures of oppression, such as gender, but also class, race, ethnicity, sexuality, nationality, and related intersectional categories."[31] In one of our interviews, an Irish legal expert described the disciplining device in the cervical cancer crisis as follows: "It would be better if victims and women in particular just shut up."

Women affected by the crisis, however, acknowledged the history of shame and silence in Ireland, drawing on this interdiction to spur them toward truth-telling and action. In response to the CervicalCheck crisis, Migrants and Ethnic-minorities for Reproductive Justice (MERJ), a group of migrants and ethnic-minorities living in Ireland fighting for reproductive justice for all people, posted: "This is outrageous! It is also important to note that migrants without PPS [Personal Public Service] numbers are not entitled to smear tests under the Cervical Check system. We must demand reproductive justice for EVERYONE in Ireland."[32] The women who brought attention to the CervicalCheck scandal faced scrutiny and public attacks to improve healthcare for all women, but they persisted in their truth-telling.

In the 2018 Scally Report, many individuals credited Vicky Phelan, who refused to sign a confidentiality clause as part of her €2.5 million court case, with highlighting the failures of CervicalCheck. Phelan was diagnosed with cervical cancer in 2014, and a routine audit found that her 2011 Pap test was incorrect. However, she was not informed about the audit until 2017. Scally described the widespread nondisclosure of standard CervicalCheck audits as a "whole-system failure." MERJ similarly called out systemic, widespread failures in its response to the CervicalCheck scandal, posting "This is why we need #ReproductiveJustice."[33] In July 2019, Professor Brian MacCraith, the President of Dublin City University, released an independent review of CervicalCheck, finding that more than 800 women and their physicians had not been informed about the results of their screening test due to information technology failings and human error. The report found a lack of clear responsibilities and authority within the CervicalCheck system. MacCraith recommended the HSE adopt a "women-first" approach to focus on providing continuous information to women, improve customer relationship management, and build trust. Succeeding in a women-first approach, however, will require a commitment to dialogic communication ethics, including truth-telling, which can repair, reconcile, and protect communities and cultures after disruption and conflict.[34]

Finally, in 2019, the UK Royal College of Obstetricians and Gynecologists (RCOG) conducted an external, independent review to better understand how many samples were misread. An expert panel reviewed 1,038 cancer slides and determined that 159 women could have been diagnosed earlier. Among those 159 cases, at least 12 women have died. At the time the report was released, there were more than 100 legal cases filed against CervicalCheck. As a result of the uncertainty surrounding CervicalCheck, women were offered a free repeat test; however, they often waited more than twenty weeks to receive their results. In an interview on RTE Radio One's *Morning Ireland*, Dr. Noirin Russell said, "It's really important not to underestimate how stressful it is for women waiting for an appointment that we're unable to tell them when it will be."[35]

Despite the flaws in the system, health providers emphasize that they believe in cervical cancer screening and its ability to prevent cervical cancer. According to Dr. Brendan O'Shea, a general practitioner in Kildare County and a member of the council at the Irish College of General Practitioners, "Regarding CervicalCheck, the science of this says we must match the courage and trust of thousands of women who attend practices for cervical screening every day and commit to do it better, while carefully remembering those who the system has failed."[36] According to an expert we interviewed from a national women's health organization in Ireland, "If you look at [CervicalCheck's] success at reducing cancer over a number of years it's really impressive . . . I think what needs to happen now is we need to restore the reputation of CervicalCheck, I think it's very important and has had a really positive impact."

In what activists described as a "watershed moment," Leo Varadkar, Taoiseach [Prime Minister], apologized for the CervicalCheck failures on behalf of the government.[37] On October 22, 2019, he said, "On behalf of the Government and the State, I am sorry it happened. And I apologize to all those hurt or wronged. And we now vow to make sure it never happens to anyone else again." He added, "We are sorry for the failures of clinical governance, sorry for the failures of leadership and management, sorry for the failure to tell the whole truth and to do so in a timely manner, sorry for the humiliation, the disrespect and deceit."[38] Advocates described the apology as "an acknowledgement from the core of our Government that our healthcare system was not patient-centered."[39] In the years since the apology, the government has worked to implement new policies to address the failings of CervicalCheck. Then–Minister for Health Simon Harris said that CervicalCheck had caused "massive pain and hurt to people right across the country" and worked to release a new patient safety bill, which ensures mandatory disclosure to patients.[40] Since March 2020, CervicalCheck now provides HPV cervical screening, which offers additional accuracy.

REVEALING TRUTH-TELLING

Through truth-telling, women revealed and confronted systems of inequality that perpetuate shame and stigma around women's bodies and health. In the Irish context, truth-telling and activism have been necessary to spur the state to take action through redress schemes. This analysis shows that the CervicalCheck scandal gained national recognition because women refused to be silent. As an expert from a national women's organization in Ireland stated in an interview with us: "What was essential to [the CervicalCheck] issue was women talking about their experiences and being unwilling to sign an NDA [nondisclosure agreement] and talking about the treatment they had and the inquiry that was commissioned into the government was saying, women are always asking why is this always happening to women in Ireland and [Scally] named issues like patriarchy in the health service." Experts and activists positioned the CervicalCheck scandal as part of a history of women's rights abuses, such as the Magdalene laundries, Mother and Baby Homes, symphysiotomies, and the Eighth Amendment. Clara Fischer argues that "shame becomes internalized, forming part of gendered, racialized, and classed subjectivities."[41] In the cervical cancer prevention crisis, Irish women's voices and narratives exposed the consequences of perpetuating shame and stigma around women's bodies.

Historically, the government has sought to remedy wrongs by compensating victims through redress schemes. According to an expert we interviewed from a national women's organization in Ireland:

> We've seen in Ireland time and time again with the Magdalene women, children in industrial schools, the state did once have a duty of care and unfortunately it does take a lot of fighting from the survivors and their supporters to see redress schemes. I don't think Ireland has gotten redress right yet and here's an opportunity where we have another chance to do that and we're not taking it. I think what people want and what so many women who were affected by the CervicalCheck scandal want, is for the screening service itself to be something people can stand over, to be trustworthy and that's a big responsibility and something the government can surely do is make sure the system is working for women.

Scholars argue that a fundamental prerequisite to trust is honesty. Another of our interview participants, a legal expert, explains:

> I think before we apply any new redress schemes, we need to have a human rights review of the habits of redress that have been developed, finessed over time by the Department of Justice and the State. We have ample evidence now to say people who participate in those schemes feel bullied, marginalized, shamed, and often regret that they accepted the redress scheme . . . Most people place more emphasis on the importance of truth-telling. I think truth-telling is an important aspect of reproductive justice

because in international human rights law, one of the key human rights guarantees is nonrepetition, and I don't think you can guarantee nonrepetition if you don't know what you did. If you don't investigate the patterns of abuse that we were complicit in the past you can't guarantee something similar won't happen in the future.

Attempts at redress have been limited by systems of social inequality that restrict women's rights. CervicalCheck shows that women's bodies and health will continue to be marginalized in a patriarchal system. In this context, redress offers limited benefits to the women impacted by CervicalCheck and fails to prevent future harm. A reproductive justice approach to reforming redress schemes must be grounded in human rights and a commitment to nonrepetition to avoid further victimization.

Moreover, redress schemes must include truth-telling, which is particularly important because attempts at redress have also attempted to silence women through nondisclosure, confidentiality clauses, sealing of records, and other methods. Scholars argue that truth-telling and resulting policies must be understood in the social, political, and historical context of the injustice.[42] Truth-telling is a form of resistance and has the potential to initiate a broader societal dialogue to define and understand human rights.[43] In Ireland, social media provided a platform for women to share their narratives of health and illness in greater numbers than ever before. For the first time, women's ways of knowing and their lived bodily experiences became central features in the national discourse. Irish women with a public platform, such as those with terminal cancer, as well as large numbers of anonymous women shared their stories to overcome the shame and stigma historically linked to women's bodies and health. Although testimonials remain vulnerable to long-standing biases and prejudices,[44] the scale and authenticity of Irish truth-telling succeeded in changing the conversation around women's health. Emily Rosser emphasizes that while advances in law are important, truth-telling, activists, and advocacy remain crucial components of establishing women's human rights.[45] The commitment of advocates over decades has been essential to providing a space for women to speak out today and spurring the state to take action through redress schemes.

In addition to the social and legal issues advanced through truth-telling, women's stories have raised cervical cancer to the national spotlight as an important health issue. According to an expert we interviewed from a national women's health organization in Ireland: "One unintended consequence of speaking out is that you can actually see that people have a name, there's someone to identify with the devastating affects cervical cancer can have. It's probably not the way you want to do health promotion campaigns but the importance of regular screening has been highlighted through that controversy." An expert from a different national women's organization concurred: "In terms of uptake, there's a positive impact because people are hearing about cervical cancer, they're hearing from women speaking about how it's impacted their lives. This is not the way to increase uptake of screening, but it has been [increasing]." The women impacted by the CervicalCheck scandal shared their stories to change the narrative around cervical cancer, personalize the issue, and save the lives of other women.

The CervicalCheck scandal bolstered a national commitment to cervical cancer screening and improved healthcare for women. According to Lorraine Walsh, who was impacted by the CervicalCheck scandal and formerly served on the CervicalCheck steering committee: "What must follow is that those in power to do so will work to establish governance structures, the oversight, the management capacity and the quality assurance checks to ensure these failures never happen again . . . Our hope now is for a time in

Ireland when no woman will ever again have cause to doubt the avail-ability or the quality of the healthcare they receive from the State."[46] Indeed, women's commitment to one another and to building a bet-ter future was highlighted once again through this crisis. An expert from a national women's organization in Ireland remarked to us:

> Women are kind and generous in thinking about women coming after them, and what they want is for the system to be safe. I've been really impressed by people who are advocating for younger women who won't be affected in the same way they were but who they feel the screening services are really important. So the government needs to support the women who have been affected but it also needs to build a trusted system again.

The CervicalCheck scandal is just one of the latest in a series of women's health scandals that have confronted Ireland's patriarchal system. By raising their voices, women who spoke out about cervical cancer became part of a legacy of truth-telling.

HPV VACCINATION MISINFORMATION CAMPAIGN

In 2010, Ireland introduced a school-based HPV vaccination pro-gram for girls ages 12 to 13, and by 2015, 86.9% of girls completed the vaccination series. In the same year, anti-vaccine lobby groups with international support distributed misinformation in Ireland through social, local, and national media and lobbied politicians against HPV vaccination. The misinformation campaign broadcast the so-called documentary *Cervical Cancer Vaccine–Is It Safe?* on national televi-sion. The film included footage from a similar broadcast in Denmark, linking it to a coordinated international anti-vaccine movement, which may have started as a series of viral videos on YouTube, that devastated vaccine confidence in Japan, Denmark, Colombia, and Ireland.[47] The so-called documentary featured parents and teens describing side effects, injuries, and long-term health issues falsely linked to the HPV vaccine. In Ireland, the campaign fueled parental concerns about vaccine safety, and by 2017, uptake of the first dose of the HPV vaccine decreased to less than 40% of girls.

The US Healthy People guidelines target an 80% vaccination rate to reduce or eliminate six HPV-related cancers. Even when countries such as Ireland initially meet this target, "unwarranted fears about HPV vaccine and the proliferation of misinformation, particularly via social media, have proven to be significant and widespread obstacles to achieving and maintaining high vaccination rates."[48] By the time it arrived in Ireland, the HPV vaccine hesitancy crisis had already led to panic in Japan, causing vaccination rates in that country to drop from approximately 70% to less than 1%,[49] and in Denmark, where rates dropped from 79% to 17%.[50] Experts estimate that the HPV vaccine misinformation campaign in Japan caused 5,000 avoidable deaths from cervical cancer.[51]

An expert we interviewed from a national women's health organization in Ireland described the HPV vaccination misinformation campaign as "fearmongering." An Irish physician said, "I couldn't believe that I was hearing such dangerous falsehoods."[52] The misinformation campaign perpetuated stigma and shame around women's bodies and sexuality, which "cannot easily be disaggregated from long-standing myths and fears about female sexuality."[53] As a result, and as mentioned, the HPV vaccination crisis revealed the biological, economic, social, and political systems that shape women's access to and decision-making about health, including cervical cancer prevention. In part, the misinformation campaign succeeded initially because of the complicated intersections of gender, race/ethnicity, socioeconomic position, immigration status, ability, sexual orientation, and age as sources of reproductive oppression. Although HPV is a ubiquitous virus, its definition as an STI led to the social construction of cervical cancer as a stigmatized disease. Social norms impact understandings of cervical cancer (and by extension HPV) tied to identity and relational meanings. In particular, cervical cancer and HPV are perceived as a disease of the "other" and are linked to what it means to be "responsible," particularly as an adolescent or young woman.[54] In other words, women believe that cervical cancer is only a risk for "other" women, particularly women who are "irresponsible."

The misinformation campaign relied on emotional manipulation targeted at the parents of young girls. For example:

> You'll often see a scare story that says—particularly a teenage girl—has had an adverse effect to this vaccination. And it'll be delivered in a very frightening way that captures your attention. It doesn't matter that the stories lack any veracity. What matters is they scare us and in scaring us we remember them. And in remembering them, we afford them more weight than they deserve. And so starts a vicious cycle. This explains why lies about the HPV vaccine were able to do so much damage in so many countries.[55]

Since mothers overwhelmingly make vaccination decisions for this children, the decision to choose the HPV vaccine for their daughters also relates to what it means to be a good mother. Scholars also argue that anti-vaccination campaigns take advantage of scientific uncertainty and lack of knowledge: "What from a scientific and public health viewpoint appears as a medical breakthrough—the creation of a drug that protects against cervical and other forms of cancer—becomes translated into a tough choice that parents must make regarding their children's future health."[56] In the context of these misinformation campaigns, parents continued striving to make the best decision for their children.

To combat the misinformation campaign, as discussed earlier, over thirty-five Irish organizations, charities, and public institutions joined together in 2017 to form the HPV Vaccination Alliance. According to a member of the HPV Vaccination Alliance we interviewed, the initiative achieved success by broadening the base of people who advocated for the vaccine, including parents:

> We're a pretty small country and community and there are a lot of people coalesced around this issue, so I think that was one of the ways we were able to combat what [the misinformation campaign] was saying. There has to be quite a lot of training with the media, not that you can train the media, but talking about the evidence, actual numbers, and new voices available to speak on the evidence. It was very much led by the cancer community but they were really good at drawing on all these other groups, who had other pieces of experience to talk about. Like so many countries, we had issues around the MMR vaccine as well, so people had experience on how to combat the antivaxxers.

The Alliance promoted HPV vaccination through a communication campaign, incorporating social and traditional media, as well as personal testimonies. Initially, health, children, and women's groups signed a Contract Against Cancer to publicly declare a commitment against misinformation. The Alliance spearheaded a #HPVVAXFACTS campaign to provide fact-based information about the HPV vaccine and HPV-caused cancers. They also created a series of videos talking with parents and cervical cancer survivors about their choice to vaccinate.

In Ireland, HPV vaccination has started to increase again, reaching approximately 61.7% in 2018[57] and approximately 75% in 2019.[58]

According to Simms and colleagues: "The events relating to HPV vaccination in Ireland and Denmark show that it is possible to reverse rapid declines in HPV vaccine coverage due to vaccine hesitancy and successfully address safety concerns reported in the media. Strong support from government is required and is most effective when there is cooperation across multiple sectors."[59] Ireland's ability to successfully counter HPV vaccine hesitancy depended on ethical communication and support from stakeholders, including partnerships between government and activists.[60]

Ethical communication must move beyond truthfulness and reliability of information toward beneficence or "the duty to contribute to a better society, to social justice, to the good of the people."[61] In particular, ethical communication aims to protect and advance the position of individuals in vulnerable situations. According to Hugo Aznar and Marcia Castillo-Martin, ethical communication intends "to give voice to those affected by a situation, and especially those in a situation of vulnerability, because this is the prime way in which they can make their voices heard and improve their situation."[62] Within this context, Vicky Phelan and other women impacted by the CervicalCheck scandal became advocates for HPV vaccination. Scholars identified "hard-hitting personal testimonials" as a key component of the HPV Vaccination Alliance's communication campaign.[63] Laura Brennan, who died from cervical cancer in March 2019, consulted about HPV advocacy for the WHO. She said, "This illness is devastating and it's going to take my life but the good news is there's a vaccine that you can get that prevents it. HPV caused my cancer. I just wanted parents to know there is an alternative."[64] Vicky Phelan wrote on Twitter, "We have a vaccine that can prevent future generations of women developing cervical cancer. As someone who is terminally ill with this cancer, I urge you to get your children vaccinated. You. Do. Not. Want. This."[65]

The truth-telling that revealed the CervicalCheck scandal became a critical feature of the HPV Vaccination Alliance's communication campaign. Experts suggest that these women's voices successfully reached parents:

> But in Ireland, what really changed the situation was a woman called Laura Brennan. When Laura was 24 she was diagnosed with cervical cancer, and by the time she was 25, that was metastatic, noncurable. Laura was alarmed that people weren't getting this vaccine that could prevent women from being in the situation that she found herself in. Her campaigning started with a series of advertisements where she talked to parents, directly to them.[66]

In a video titled, "Don't Be Swayed by Rumors," aimed at parents, Laura discussed her cervical cancer diagnosis and treatment, sharing that when her cancer returned, there was no treatment that could cure her cancer. She said, "If anything good comes out of this, I would hope parents would get their daughters vaccinated. The vaccine saves lives, it could have saved mine."[67]

The central lesson of the HPV vaccination misinformation campaign reflects the crucial need to listen: "It is incumbent on experts involved in medical and scientific risk communication to be alert and sensitive to the side effects of uncertainty and its capacity to generate anxiety."[68] According to Hugo Aznar and Marcia Castillo-Martin, ethical communication must "be oriented to make the participation of the people easier, to promote their sense of being a part of the public debate, a part of the social community in dialogue."[69] The success of the HPV Vaccination Alliance is promising as Ireland works to modernize healthcare and serve the needs of women; however, the threat has not been eradicated: "A combination of hard-hitting personal testimonials, social media and traditional media promoted the

HPV vaccine. Despite this, systematic engagement and supranational strategies are still in the early stages of being formulated. As misleading information spreads through social media and digital networks have undesirable impacts on attitudes to vaccination (and uptake rates), urgent actions are required."[70]

CONCLUSION: A WOMEN-FIRST APPROACH

CervicalCheck and the HPV vaccination misinformation campaign revealed institutionalized misogyny within Ireland's government, healthcare system, and society. As an expert from a national women's organization in Ireland said to us, "The reality is most of the health services in Ireland have been religious ones and that has impacted so many services like symphysiotomy and all these areas that a moralistic approach to sexuality has been very clear for women." In an interview with CNN, Dr. Mary McAuliffe, historian in Gender Studies at University College Dublin, described how this approach to sexuality has impacted women's health: "Women's bodies and the risk to women's bodies are not important—and in particular their reproductive bodies and their healthcare is seen as secondary to maybe money, to power, and to a patriarchal system that has always seen women as second class citizens."[71] Despite a system that has historically devalued them, women continue to engage in story-telling about health, illness, and the body to confront, challenge, and change Ireland's healthcare system.

The 2018 Scally Report and the 2019 MacCraith Review[72] recommended a women-first approach to healthcare. In a Twitter thread, Vicky Phelan responded to these recommendations:

Dr Scally recommended that the Minister of Health Simon Harris "give consideration to how women's health issues can be given more consistent, expert and committed attention" within our health system. Professor MacCraith has recommended a "Women First" approach. WE NEED TO MAKE THIS HAPPEN.

We need to take women's health more seriously. Dr Scally demanded that "more and different attention NEEDS to be paid to women's health issues". It is simply not enough to pay lip service to women's health. We have had enough.[73]

Cliona Loughnane of the National Women's Council shared a similar sentiment about what needs to happen next: "We need to put structures in place and the policies in place that react to what women say they need on the ground."[74]

Listening to women may be the best way to improve healthcare. According to an interview we conducted with an expert on women's health, "I think what the CervicalCheck scandal showed is that we need as much attention on women's health, on taking it seriously." In order to take women's health seriously, the practices that emerge must focus on truth-telling as an important aspect of reproductive justice. Ethical communication about cervical screening is a first step toward this goal, as another expert, from a national women's organization, expressed:

> The [patient involvement] panel we're on is about the information going out to women on cervical screening and about open disclosure and consent, so there's a real attempt to let women know what screenings can pick up and what screenings cannot pick up, what you're consenting to, and so on. That's being done in this new modern way of helping healthcare and helping get information to patients is providing women with expertise on women's health.

Ultimately, a women-first approach to healthcare must be grounded in ethical communication. Indeed, "social communication has to be a way to build an effective community through the communicative participation of the individuals."[75]

Patriarchy in the health service emerged as a primary cause of the cervical cancer prevention crisis. The ongoing impact of Ireland's religious health services was evident in the CervicalCheck scandal and the HPV vaccination misinformation campaign. Patriarchy and religious health services impacted the care women received related to HPV vaccination and cervical cancer screening by perpetuating a moral approach to female sexuality grounded in myths and fear of women. Women themselves, however, challenged these systems through truth-telling. Through advocacy and raising their voices, women contested medical authority. They addressed issues of consent, the right to knowledge about their own bodies, and scientific uncertainty. Finally, as Ireland strives toward a women-first approach to healthcare, experts argue that reforming redress schemes must be grounded in human rights and a commitment to nonrepetition to avoid further victimization. Overcoming misogyny will depend on listening to women and addressing shame and stigma around women's bodies.

Although gains have been made, advocates continue to identify flaws in Ireland's commitment to nonrepetition. In October 2020, the CervicalCheck Tribunal was established as an alternative legal mechanism, outside of the court, to hear and determine claims from the CervicalCheck scandal. The goal is for the Tribunal to be expeditious, effective, and less adversarial than the court. However, CervicalCheck campaigners, including Vicky Phelan, have expressed concerns about the Tribunal, including the statute of limitations and the issue of cancer recurrence. The proposed 2019 Patient Safety Bill, which would provide open disclosure and mandatory reporting of serious patient safety incidents, is still being amended and debated in 2023 despite the government confirming its commitment to the legislation. Although truth-telling has demonstrably improved cervical cancer prevention in Ireland, the CervicalCheck Tribunal and Patient Safety Bill provide evidence that challenges to achieving reproductive justice remain.

Ethical communication is evident in the success of the HPV Vaccination Alliance in restoring confidence in the HPV vaccine. Still, gaps in ethical communication in Ireland emerge regarding Traveller, refugee, and asylum-seeking women. For example, in the context of the cervical cancer scandal, MERJ reminded advocates on social media that migrants without Personal Public Service (PPS) numbers are not entitled to smear tests through CervicalCheck. Truth-telling offers one approach to elevating discord in social media advocacy by emphasizing accountability to women's voices, avoiding reifying or essentializing women's experiences, and affirming local women's meaning making.[76] In response to Ireland's cervical cancer prevention crisis, advocates embraced digital intersectional communication through a reproductive justice approach to truth-telling.

This study revealed social constructions and attitudes toward gender and women's health in Ireland. Applying a reproductive justice lens to the cervical cancer prevention crisis revealed the importance of truth-telling as a form of resistance and empowering women to make decisions about their own bodies through a women-first approach to healthcare. Experts situated CervicalCheck and the HPV vaccination misinformation campaign in Ireland's patriarchal history of women's rights abuses, including the Magdalene laundries, Mother and Baby Homes, symphysiotomies, and the Eighth Amendment. By raising women's voices, advocates engaged in truth-telling about health, illness, and the body to confront, challenge, and change Ireland's healthcare system. In order to achieve reproductive justice, as well as understanding and consensus on fundamental human rights, truth-telling remains essential.

Contraception

In January 2023, the Irish government began to guarantee free contraception for women between the ages of 17 and 26.[1] This development came several years after the 2019 Report of the Working Group on Access to Contraception's recommendations, which pointed out Ireland's comparatively low contraceptive usage and identified cost, embarrassment, and ignorance as central obstacles.[2] Irish law has allowed for the purchase and use of contraceptives in most circumstances for decades, and emergency contraception has been available without a prescription since 2011. However, Ireland has one of the lowest rates of contraceptive use in the European Union.[3] The Irish case, then, points to the limits of a purely legalistic perspective, foregrounding the need for a broader, reproductive justice approach to contraceptive use, one that recognizes women's everyday embodied experiences.

Most of the focus of reproductive health in Ireland in the past few years, particularly during and after the 2018 referendum, has been on abortion; indeed, the struggle over abortion legality sometimes has curtailed the attention given to other essential issues, such as birth control. Irish activists and ordinary women, however, have consistently pushed for a comprehensive view of fertility and fertility control, including contraception, and for linking contraception and

Catching Fire. Beth Sundstrom and Cara Delay, Oxford University Press. © Oxford University Press 2023.
DOI: 10.1093/oso/9780197743942.003.0003

abortion as two related and essential elements of bodily autonomy. As one activist told us:

> A free safe legal abortion is made less common if you have free, safe, effective contraception, and so in a constrained healthcare system, contraception should be free, in fact all contraception should be free. Women should have the full choice of what they want to use, as they do in many other jurisdictions, for example in the UK.... It's just not as sexy as repeal the 8th! Free condoms for everybody! It's less of a campaign thing, and I get that, but it's essential.

An obstetrician we interviewed discussed how the abortion Repeal campaign foregrounded the need for long-acting reversible contraception (LARC) in Ireland:

> The Irish Pharmacy Association wanted to put something in [the abortion legislation] about having hormonal contraception available at pharmacies. So pharmacists could provide these options, and in reaction to that, the Irish Family Planning Association said we should put something in about long-lasting reversible contraception and an emphasis on IUDs [intrauterine devices] and implants. I'm interested in how the repeal and legislation may impact other areas of women's health as well.

Similarly, the narratives publicized via digital activism link contraception and abortion, making birth control a central part of the conversation on bodily autonomy. Contributors to *In Her Shoes*, a platform created on Facebook and Twitter in 2018 to facilitate women's anonymous abortion story-telling, pointed out that their need for abortion sometimes stemmed from contraceptive failure, physicians' reluctance to prescribe birth control, ignorance about birth control, or problems accessing contraception.[4]

This chapter explores how health activists, feminist organizations, and women posting on social media have worked to increase knowledge and use of contraception in Ireland via truth-telling: by dispelling birth control myths, combatting contraceptive ignorance and opposition, and sharing everyday embodied realities. It assesses the obstacles to contraceptive access, confronting misconceptions and establishing birth control as an essential element of women's overall health and well-being within the larger movement for reproductive justice. The government's recent attempts to study contraceptive usage and move toward greater access have begun to succeed because of the roles played by ordinary activists and activist movements—often across decades—in bringing issues associated with contraception to the public's attention. This chapter positions contraception as an urgent need in Ireland today that must be addressed within the framework of reproductive justice and achieved through truth-telling and by foregrounding the experiences of people who need and want birth control.

REPRODUCTIVE JUSTICE AND CONTRACEPTION

A 2010 study based on a nationwide survey revealed that 16% of pregnancies in the Republic of Ireland were crisis pregnancies, defined as unplanned or mistimed.[5] Of those women experiencing crisis pregnancies, "use of no contraception and use of poor efficacy contraception methods were cited as the most common contraceptive methods used at the time of conception of the crisis pregnancy." Strikingly, almost 60% of respondents to the 2010 survey claimed that they were not using any form of contraception before their crisis pregnancy.[6] Moreover, approximately one-third of Irish women who completed a survey several years later, in 2014, reported not using any type of birth control; responding to the survey, Dr. Shirley McQuade, director of Dublin's Well Woman Centre, said:

> I'm surprised such a high number of women in Ireland are not using any contraception. Even when you remove those women who are planning on having a child this year (13 per cent), that still leaves one woman in five (20 per cent) who are neither using contraception nor planning on getting pregnant within the year.[7]

This same study also revealed that only 46% of women believed that contraception was a shared responsibility between them and their partner. For women, accessing and using reliable birth control remains a significant responsibility and a significant issue today.

A health activist we interviewed in 2018 described the obstacles to birth control usage in Ireland:

> I meet a lot of people with unplanned pregnancies and it's just lack of knowledge, people do not know how to use or take the pill properly, they don't. Either they can't afford it, they think they don't need it, there's a lack of education amongst young people as to what constitutes you, what kind of makes a baby and what doesn't. . . . Young women learn from each other, and they're not necessarily giving the correct information. . . . and they're all saying the same lies so they're all kind of teaching each other, you know?

This participant identified ignorance as one of the most significant barriers to effective contraceptive use. Most studies affirm this, suggesting that Irish people's knowledge and understanding of birth control and contraceptive methods, although improving, lag behind those of their European peers. A 2020 survey by the Well Woman Centre asked Irish women between the ages of 17 and 45 about their understandings of contraceptive use and efficacy. The results revealed that between 49% and 53% of women did not know the failure rates of the birth control pill and condoms (9% and 17%, respectively, based on typical use). Moreover, 10% of those surveyed believed that the withdrawal method was an effective form of pregnancy preven- tion, while 21% erroneously thought that "you can't get pregnant if you have sex during your period."[8]

Other evidence points to ignorance about the interactions between certain medications and the birth control pill. In 2018, for example, an anonymous woman posted to *In Her Shoes*: "My birth control failed while taking antibiotics, I never even thought about antibiotics making the pill less effective. To say the pregnancy was a shock is an understatement."[9] The following narrative, told to us by a Repeal activist, reminds us that ignorance about birth control is endemic in Irish society and affects all people, not just women: "One time a man came up to the stall one day, because people prepared their [abortion rights] speeches, and he said 'you've been asking for contraception since the 70s, and now you've got it and you won't use it,' and I said to him 'did you know that contraception fails?' and he was like oh, what?"

The issue of contraceptive ignorance may stem, in part, from the reality that birth control was legalized relatively late in Ireland—in the 1970s and 1980s—as well as the pervasive culture of silence— what Tom Inglis calls "the old Catholic-church strategy of not referring directly to sex and sexuality"—that persisted until recent decades.[10] Intimately related to this cultural ignorance is embar- rassment. Twenty-five percent of Irish respondents who described obstacles to accessing contraception in 2010 cited embarrass- ment as a key factor.[11] Similarly, the government's 2019 Report of the Working Group on Access to Contraception found that young women felt embarrassed accessing contraception, including "being afraid to reveal they are sexually active; embarrassed to be seen at a family planning clinic; or worried about confidentiality breaches."[12] One woman described what happened when, as a teenager, she asked her mother about birth control. Her mother's response was that she "wouldn't allow it, as good catholic [sic] girls don't have sex and the shame I would bring if she had to ask the doctor."[13]

Clara Fischer's recent work has explored the historical and cultural origins of embarrassment and its deeper, more insidious companion, shame. In discussing what she calls "a politics of shame," Fischer links the persistent shame and embarrassment related to Irish sexuality and bodies to the nation's postcolonial identity formation, arguing that in the early twentieth century, the newly independent Ireland positioned "women's sexuality and bodies as problematic, potentially sinful, and in need of control lest the nation's very identity be put at risk."[14] The historical regulation of women's sexuality and bodies through forced migration, institutionalization, and legal restrictions on abortion and contraception is well known.[15] Even after some of these restrictions were lifted or institutions closed, however, the shame that was their constant companion persisted, manifesting in the embarrassment that some women felt, and continue to feel, when attempting to access contraception—and, thus, potentially expose themselves as sexual beings and bodies.

Certain marginalized groups in Ireland, including migrant and Traveller women, may have even less access to and knowledge of contraception. Ireland's migrant population has swelled in recent years; the decade from 1996 to 2006 witnessed a threefold increase in migrants into the country.[16] Ronit Lentin points out the racism and sexism with which the government has responded to large numbers of specifically migrant women, many of childbearing age, in Ireland.[17] "Those whose bodies are excluded from the borders of citizenship," writes Katherine Side, "may experience limitations in access and/or are more likely to be subjected to state regulatory bodies and scrutiny."[18]

Studies of migrant women have found levels of contraceptive ignorance comparable to those of nonmigrant women; migrant women, however, often face additional challenges accessing contraception, including communication struggles. According to a 2014 report by the website sexualwellbeing.ie:

> [Migrant] women reported low levels of engagement with Irish health services due to language issues, limited knowledge of services and unfamiliarity with how to access services. Pharmacies were often cited as a key source of information and advice on health issues. Some women used websites to get contraceptives.[19]

Some migrant women concerned with the cost of birth control in Ireland "bought contraceptive products from pharmacies and doctors in their home countries, sometimes 'bulk buying' to try to ensure they had what they needed."[20] Others periodically traveled to their country of origin to access healthcare and obtain contraception. A 25-year-old Chinese national, Ying, told researchers:

> YING: So I think for most crisis pregnancies girls don't know this would happen to you and you always think it's someone else's story and you wouldn't think it would happen to you. And honestly I felt awkward as well, a reason why there would be crisis pregnancies as well, I felt awkward to go get the contraception so I would go back home once a year and because condoms were cheaper back home I'd . . .
> INTERVIEWER: Stock up?
> YING: Yeah![21]

These realities mean that some of these women do not establish relationships with physicians in Ireland and, if they need contraception, emergency contraception, and/or abortion care while in Ireland, are consequently disadvantaged. In addition, for young unmarried migrant women, social and familial pressures can be particularly powerful, affecting their access to reproductive healthcare services. A 2012 Health Service Executive (HSE) study on migrant women revealed:

> Migrant families are expected to progress and succeed in their new country, and so a young woman becoming pregnant is a greater "failure" when those "back home" are considered: failure by her to optimise enhanced educational opportunities in her new country of residence and failure by her family to maintain the moral standards of their "old" country of origin. This creates particular conditions for the possibility of crisis pregnancy among young migrant women.[22]

In some migrant communities, young women are expected to refrain from sex until marriage; therefore, discussions about birth control are lacking. This same study demonstrated that young unmarried migrant women found it difficult to access contraception and expressed some resistance to using hormonal contraception.[23]

Activist group AkiDwA ("sisterhood" in Swahili), founded in 1999, has consistently worked to improve healthcare access for migrant women in Ireland. AkiDwA's 2017 study divulged that

> many women feel there is a lack of understanding of their cultural background and country of origin from the healthcare providers, resulting in misunderstandings, negative perspectives and stereotypes, which then in turn hinder equality and integration.[24]

Girls and women living in Direct Provision, the system that houses asylum-seekers in Ireland, appear to be particularly vulnerable. A 2019 report compiled by the Irish Family Planning Association (IFPA) focused on the difficulties that people in Direct Provision have accessing reproductive healthcare:

> In our experience, women living in Direct Provision are frequently unaware of: free screening programmes such as CervicalCheck and BreastCheck; the availability of abortion services and different methods of long-term contraception; and where and how to seek treatment for sexually transmitted infections and issues relating to menopause, fertility and menstruation.[25]

Ireland's ethnic minority Traveller community faces its own unique struggles accessing healthcare. Travellers "form a small indigenous ethnic minority set apart from the settled population by distinctive cultural values, language and nomadic tradition, and they have much in common with European Travellers and Gypsies."[26] The long history of state-endorsed racism against Travellers and a lack of research, until recently, about their healthcare needs have resulted in a lack of data about their contraceptive use. A significant study conducted in 2003, however, found that Traveller women's use of birth control is significantly lower than that of non-Traveller women.[27] Like migrant women, Traveller women face issues accessing and communicating with healthcare providers, with their needs and wants often dismissed. One woman, speaking of medical professionals, told researchers "most of them treated us Travellers like nobodies . . . didn't want to take time to speak to us. The doctors and nurses don't understand and don't want to understand!"[28] Moreover, as Bernadette Reid and Julie Taylor observe, "Traveller women's divergence from the presumed majority 'norms' has predisposed them to a politics of victim-blaming, in which cultural attributes are regarded as different and pathological."[29] For example, the tendency amongst some Traveller women to marry and reproduce at younger ages than the settled population may result in a dismissal of their contraceptive needs.

These complex realities remind us about the importance of analyzing contraception within a reproductive justice framework, placing birth control within the contexts of education, knowledge, and access and through an intersectional lens that considers race or ethnicity, religion, region, sexuality, and socioeconomic position. Reproductive justice scholars underscore access to birth control as essential, encouraging us to look beyond legality to examine "the social context in which individuals live and make their personal decisions."[30] An elemental aspect of this context is women's economic circumstances. Indeed, alongside ignorance and embarrassment, cost has been identified as one of the most significant barriers to birth control use in Ireland. In June 2021, the *Irish Medical Journal* published a study revealing that "unreliable" and "inconsistent" contraceptive use rates among Irish university students could be explained, in part, by cost. Providing lower-cost or free birth control, the study's authors argued, would not only increase contraceptive usage but also encourage both women and men to explore different methods, perhaps moving from the currently popular, but less reliable, condoms, the pill, and coitus interruptus to more effective LARC methods.[31]

Activists and healthcare professionals we interviewed consistently affirmed that cost remained a significant barrier to contraceptive access in Ireland. As one told us:

Well the most pressing [obstacle] is cost, because you know, if you're in your 20's, and you're not in college, and don't have a medical card, you're talking about potentially paying 60 euro to go to a GP [general practitioner], minimum. And then your pill prescription on top of that, so you're kind of . . . if you're on a cheap pill every 3 months which people just don't have.

In the Republic of Ireland, the costs of birth control vary based on both contraceptive method and the status of the user. Just over 30% of the population has a government-issued medical card, which allows them access to low-cost contraception, including some LARC methods. For those who do not hold a medical card, however, the costs are much higher: approximately €250 to €350 for most LARC methods.[32] For those without a medical card, the birth control pill can also be prohibitively expensive. A recent study found that "18.8% of oral contraception users without a medical card had missed taking the pill because they could not afford the prescription."[33]

Women who posted to *In Her Shoes* identified the cost of various contraceptive methods as significant obstacles to pregnancy prevention. As one woman related:

My cycle was always exactly the same each month, so I decided to plan around the days pre and ovulation with condoms while saving up to get the copper coil. This method worked perfectly for months. One month my period was late, which is strange and is usually due to stress. I took a pregnancy the day after I was due, which showed negative. I continued to do one every day of that week, and still negative every time. I put it down to coming off contraceptive after 5 years or to stress. After 2 weeks when I still had no period I decided to double check. And there it was, I was pregnant.[34]

This woman's inability to afford a reliable IUD led to a preventable crisis pregnancy, and many women have faced similar circumstances in Ireland. A 2021 study that interviewed university students in

Ireland exposed that the most popular methods of birth control—condoms, the birth control pill, and coitus interruptus—were chosen primarily because of cost. In fact, 39% of women interviewed in the study claimed that they would change contraceptive methods, considering the coil (as IUDs are often called in Ireland) or implant, if cost were not an issue.[35]

HISTORY AND TRUTH-TELLING

Truth-telling is necessary in order to combat the ignorance, embarrassment, and shame related to contraception as well as the economic obstacles that many people face in accessing birth control. Notably, however, public campaigns and government messaging on contraception remain rare. As an obstetrician/gynecologist activist told us in 2018 when asked about campaigns on contraception:

> I really can't think of anything, which isn't good is it? I'm trying to think of posters or anything . . . um, no. There's actually genuinely nothing coming to mind. Maybe if I sat down and really thought about it, but nothing is really coming to mind. . . . I suppose in our hospital we're kind of providing more verbal information, we don't really have, there wouldn't be a big drive for contraception advertising in a maternity hospital. Except for, kind of when I'm in the emergency room . . . we don't have to, it's not really one of our most pressing campaigns.

The government's 2019 Report of the Working Group on Access to Contraception was an attempt to improve communication on birth control access and usage. The report also highlighted the government's earlier attempts to address contraception with the Crisis Pregnancy Agency (now the HSE Sexual Health and Crisis Pregnancy Programme (SHCPP)) established almost 20 years ago in 2001. . . . In relation to Sexual and Reproductive Health (SRH) more generally, the National Sexual Health Strategy (2015–2020) is being implemented to improve sexual health and well-being and reduce negative sexual health outcomes. This Strategy, launched on 29th October 2015, represents the first time that a nationally coordinated approach had been developed to address sexual health and wellbeing in Ireland.[36]

Also significant to the 2019 Report was the 2017 recommendation of the Citizens' Assembly on the Eighth Amendment, a government-appointed group tasked with considering the future of the anti-abortion Eighth Amendment. The Citizens' Assembly report, surprisingly to many, linked contraception and abortion, stating: "Improved access to reproductive healthcare services should be available to all women—to include family planning services, contraception, perinatal hospice care and termination of pregnancy if required."[37]

These government strategies and initiatives, however, must combat negative media reporting on contraception, or "contraceptive scare." Some media outlets perpetuate scaremongering in terms of birth control, emphasizing or overstating the potentially adverse healthcare effects of using hormonal contraception.[38] Women interviewed in Galway, Ireland, in 2014 demonstrated the results of such tactics: 37% of those interviewed expressed concerns about allegedly dangerous side effects of the birth control pill, which, they claimed, made them reluctant to use it.[39] In 1995, the United Kingdom, Germany, and the Netherlands preemptively (before studies were peer reviewed and published) warned physicians of the blood-clot risks that new-generation birth control pills posed to women.[40] Although the Irish Medical Board did not issue similar warnings, the United Kingdom's caution was reported on extensively in Ireland, resulting in lower use of the birth control pill there.[41] In recent decades, the advent of digital media, including Facebook, Twitter, and YouTube, has had a complicated effect: on the one hand, such platforms have facilitated a more democratized participation in media; on the other hand, scaremongering and "quack" science have been able to reach a much larger audience.[42]

Although current research on contraceptive scare in Ireland is lacking, scholarship on similar topics in other Western countries is informative. Studies of social media have shown that "hormono-phobia," defined as fear or suspicion of "all forms of hormonal con-traception: pills, patches, rings, injectables, implants and hormonal intrauterine devices (IUDs)," is pervasive, brought about, in part, by an overemphasis on social media of the health risks associated with such methods. Moreover, in twelve studies conducted in the 2010s, some "participants characterized hormonal contraception as 'unnat-ural' or nonhormonal methods as more 'natural,' and stated that syn-thetic hormones are chemicals."[43] Despite the fact that the hormonal birth control pill is one of the most-studied and safest medications we have—safer than aspirin, in fact, as a well-known 1993 journal article stated—many social media users share their stories of "pill misery" and advocate quitting hormonal birth control.[44] A 2014 study conducted in Galway reported "misconceptions about LARCs, such as 'infertility' or 'delayed conception.'" As the creators of the study explain, "The women didn't like the idea of 'something long-term in their bodies' and 'felt more in control' using the OCP [oral contraceptive pill]. Conversations about 'horror stories' or bad expe-riences of LARCs through their social networks or the media were central to their choices."[45]

In Ireland, the legal prohibitions on contraception, which was only made available to most women in the 1980s, also have impacted attitudes toward it. An activist we interviewed in 2018 about contraception framed the current state of birth control in Ireland as a process of "catching up" to account for a restrictive past: "We had a lot of catching up to do very fast, like in 1990 you couldn't buy a condom in Ireland, it's crazy how behind we were for so long so, we had a lot of catching up to do very fast." As this activist recognized, Ireland's unique history has impacted popular impressions of, and use of, birth control today. Grappling with, and exposing, that history is an essential step in the truth-telling process.

Ireland was indeed "behind" when it came to contraceptive use throughout the twentieth century. The island's complicated twentieth century saw revolution and war from 1916 to 1923, partition in 1922 and independence for some counties, and the subsequent development of two states on one island. After partition, the independent Free State, comprising twenty-six counties outside of Ulster,[46] set about defining itself. Like many postcolonial states, the new Ireland was determined to distinguish itself from the former colonizer—Britain, in this case. During late nineteenth- and early twentieth-century nationalist movements, proponents of Home Rule or independence constructed the idea of an Ireland that would be based on "traditional" rural Gaelic culture and gender norms and distinguished from Britain via religion. Irish nationalist leaders postindependence thus set about creating a state that was defined as Catholic and based on Catholic moral teaching. For several decades after partition, "a combination of political ideology and religion effectively contracted Irish women's political role," defining them as domestic and regulating their sexuality.[47] While unmarried women were instructed to have no sexual contact whatsoever, with devastating consequences for those who did not comply, married women were encouraged to reproduce as much as possible; indeed, reproduction was declared to be their national duty.[48]

Birth control in the new, independent Catholic Ireland was framed as a moral rather than a medical issue.[49] In 1926, the government's Report of the Committee on Evil Literature problematized "the indiscriminate advertisement and circulation in Ireland of books and pamphlets advocating the use of unnatural means for the prevention of contraception."[50] Archives of the committee's deliberations and correspondence reveal discussions about having the postal service seize "obscene" materials, including advertisements on contraception.[51] In 1935, the Criminal Law Amendment Act made the importing and sale of contraceptives illegal.[52] According to Sandra McAvoy, this was a key turning point, in that it publicly declared the new Ireland to be distinct from an increasingly socially and sexually liberal Britain.[53]

By the early 1960s, the approval of the birth control pill in the United States and parts of Europe for contraceptive use promised a transformation in women's reproductive decision-making and sexual experiences, but Ireland again traveled a different path. The papal encyclical *Humanae Vitae* (1968) affirmed the Catholic Church's anti–birth control stance; this action strengthened some Catholic Irish physicians' and politicians' opposition to contraceptive liberalization.[54] It was not until 1979 that some contraceptives were decriminalized in Ireland, the same year that Irish Minister for Justice Patrick Cooney gave a speech in which he articulated: "Making contraceptives freely available in this country would be detrimental to the general good of the population."[55] And birth control without a prescription was difficult to access even through the 1980s.

In 1983, the Eighth Amendment to the Irish Constitution banned abortions unless multiple doctors determined that the pregnant person's life was in danger. However, the Eighth Amendment negatively affected women's access to vital healthcare beyond abortion. It upheld and enhanced the authority of physicians, maintaining and exacerbating hierarchies and distance between women and healthcare providers. It bolstered the pro-fertility ethos of the nation and made open discussions about accessing birth control even more difficult. Some women who used social media to discuss their experiences with contraception under the atmosphere created by the Eighth Amendment articulated these difficulties. They referenced the power of physicians and the coercive practices they faced.

Several women specifically mentioned wanting sterilization but confronting physician opposition. One posted: "From my first antenatal visit, until my last, I requested a tubular ligation. 'We'll need your husband to sign a permission slip' 'Excuse me?!' 'Oh, haha, I mean a consent form!' "[56] In Ireland, "sterilization (i.e., tubal ligation and vasectomies) is accessible on discriminatory grounds, such as 'where the family is complete.' "[57] In order to access sterilization in Ireland, women must be referred to a gynecologist by their GP, who may recommend counseling prior to offering a referral. In addition, a GP can refuse to refer a woman for sterilization if they do not believe it is in her "best interests."[58] Historical and cultural "values," biomedical power, and enhanced physician authority continue to affect Irish people's views on, and use of, birth control today. For example, a Polish migrant woman expressed her negative experiences with healthcare after moving to Ireland. She "described how when she moved to a new rural locality in the south of Ireland she attended the GP assigned to her there under the GMS [government-run medical service] for a prescription for hormonal contraception, only to discover the GP refused on conscientious objection grounds."[59]

Even young Irish adults express a lack of knowledge about birth control that stems from an inadequate, or even nonexistent, sex education. Religious beliefs that abstinence before marriage was the only option meant that until recently, sex was not taught in public schools or churches. Similarly, many parents proved unwilling to discuss anything related to sex or bodies, including fertility control, with their children.[60] A 2010 national study reported that only two-thirds of Irish parents talked about sexuality with their children.[61]

A reproductive justice approach is useful here because it considers not only legal contexts but also examines other real-world circumstances linked to birth control, including the continued problems some women have with silence and negative popular attitudes toward birth control. For younger unmarried women, the expectation that pregnancy would not occur until marriage was, and in some cases remains, stalwart. "Growing up in a family where we were all told 'if you come home pregnant, you'll be shown the door,'" a contributor to *In Her Shoes* wrote, "it was something we all laughed at and thought nothing of. Until the unthinkable happens."[62] Another woman contributed the following to *In Her Shoes*: "Coming from a very Catholic family in a rural town in Ireland meant that going to the family (male) doctor for the pill wasn't an option for me."[63] And a third similarly expressed her family's opposition to premarital sexual activity, writing: "I was 15 years old and doing what a lot of girls my age were doing i was in a relationship which i thought was love. we decided to take it to the next step been careful everytime. we would go to the shops to by condoms to make sure we were safe i couldn't ask my parents to be put on birth control (nor sure i even fully understood it)."[64] According to this contributor's account, ignorance and her parents' opposition to birth control combined, ultimately resulting in an unwanted pregnancy.

In these narratives, some women linked their experiences and ignorance with that of their mothers and grandmothers, shedding light on continuities across generations. One woman, writing of her own struggles with bodily autonomy, referenced her mother's similar circumstances years earlier: "So, in this good catholic country where our hospitals are 'overseen' by these 'good Catholic' people my mother had no choice but to continue with her pregnancy all the while getting sicker and sicker."[65] The cycle of ignorance persisted across generations and across decades of enormous social, cultural, and economic change.

Prohibitions on birth control in twentieth-century Ireland, however, should not blind us to the reality that the practices of ordinary Irish Catholics frequently dissented from the official Church stance.[66] By 1966, for example, 15,000 Irish women were taking the pill as birth control under the guise of needing to regulate their menstrual cycles.[67] Although statistics are hard to come by, hundreds of people in the 1960s also traveled to Northern Ireland to purchase contraceptives, which were legal there.[68] Nor should we forget that a significant activist movement attempted to combat the Church-state consensus and bring greater birth control access to Ireland. Laura Kelly's recent work, for example, has affirmed the important, yet often overlooked, work of feminist groups such as the Irish Women's Liberation Movement (IWLM), Irish Women United (IWU), and Contraception Action Program (CAP) in the 1970s. In the early 1970s, the IWLM, Kelly demonstrates, criticized Ireland's prohibitions on birth control but also problematized the growing global emphasis on the pill as the current form of birth control choice for women, arguing for greater contraceptive choices and options.[69] In 1975, the IWU took a more deliberate stance, linking contraceptive choice and availability to women's liberation more broadly. Meanwhile, CAP, a subgroup of the IWU, went so far in 1976 as to set up Contraceptives Unlimited, an illegal, underground shop providing nonmedical forms of birth control.[70]

Linda Connolly's work on Irish feminism cautions us to resist the tendency to present Irish women as "passive or tangential subjects in sociohistorical change," powerless in the face of the powerful patriarchal forces that structured their lives, or as "late bloomers" in terms of feminist activism. During both the first and second waves of the global feminist movement, she reminds us, women were not only powerful activists for change within Ireland but also maintained strong trans-national feminist connections.[71] Moreover, women organized for change in groups, such as the Irish Housewives' Association and the Irish Countrywoman's Association, that did not necessarily adopt an overtly feminist platform.[72] As early as the 1920s, furthermore, Irish women and men engaged in ordinary activism by writing to Marie Stopes, birth control advocate and creator of birth control clinics in the United Kingdom (including Belfast), for advice about contra-ception, and in the late 1960s, the periodical *Women's Way* featured numerous letters from Irish women inquiring about birth control.[73]

A key moment of feminist activism and resistance related to con-traception came in 1971, when nearly fifty members of the IWLM travelled to Belfast to purchase birth control (which was legal there), bringing it back, via the train, to Dublin (where it was illegal). These activists made a public splash, confronting customs officials and engaging with the media. Indeed, "the event they staged was cap-tured by photographers and filmed by TV crews from all over the world,"[74] publicizing Ireland's anti–birth control stance as well as how ordinary women were resisting it. These activists, and many others throughout the second half of the twentieth century, created a prec-edent for future activist methods that would help not only bring birth control access to the attention of the government but also overturn the Eighth Amendment in 2018. Their methods, featuring ordinary women, mass action, claiming of space, and utilizing the media, were taken up and built upon by later advocates.

Research demonstrates that despite the ignorance and misinfor-mation about contraception that persists in Ireland, the work of activ-ists and healthcare advocates is making a difference. A 2012 study focusing on migrant women found that many received information about contraception via the internet, but some knew about clinics. As an 18-year-old Muslim migrant told researchers:

M: Mhmm. There's one near the Ha'penny bridge. It's called the Women's Centre and there's another on Dame Street as well. That's two in town that women can go to and seek help. So there definitely is.

INTERVIEWER: And do you think they do good work out there?

M: Yeah, definitely. From what I've heard they do good work and promote safe sex. And there's a service where they provide counseling as well and they support women. Somebody with unplanned pregnancy, they'll give them information, they'll give them flyers and talk to a counsellor.[75]

Social media has allowed women to give voice to "topics and experiences that were common historically (and recently) but rarely recognized both by Irish society and by scholars."[76] Katherine Side writes that during the Repeal campaign of 2018, "Story-telling permitted individuals to reshape their own narratives and allowed them to counter stereotypes about sexual morality, contraceptive carelessness, and the extent to which pregnancy loss was or was not mourned. Individuals asserted agency for their own decision-making through stories."[77] Women who utilized social media became ordinary activists, engaging in truth-telling to combat the shame and silences that continue to affect women's health, including contraceptive use, in Ireland today.

BIRTH CONTROL METHODS

In the Republic of Ireland today, a majority of birth control users utilize two particular methods: the birth control pill and condoms.[78] These methods, however, are less reliable and more subject to individual misuse than long-acting reversible contraception (LARC) methods, including the IUD and implant. In 2015, IUDs accounted for only 7.5% of birth control use in Irish women, and this percentage was even lower for younger women.[79]

According to Dublin's Well Woman Centre, 35% of women surveyed in 2020 who experienced contraceptive failure faced an unexpected pregnancy.[80] Indeed, several contributors to *In Her Shoes* described crisis pregnancies after the pill or condoms failed (or were misused). In April 2018, one woman living in Direct Provision wrote:

> I came to Ireland 3 years ago with my 2 kids because where we were living was not safe for us. Now we live in a small room together in a Direct Provision center. I have been taking birth control pills because I don't want to have more children while we have to live in this place. Direct Provision is no place for children. They have no place to play, especially when it is cold and raining outside. I didn't think I would become pregnant because I was taking my pills everyday, but then I missed my period. I took a pregnancy test and it was positive.[81]

Numerous other postings similarly described the failure of the birth control pill and condom:

> It was about 7 years ago, I was 23, my boyfriend of 2 years at the time was 29. We lived together, we both had jobs, my boyfriend worked in a bar at night and I was a couple of months in to my first employed full-time career job since graduating from university. I was on the pill at the time, and had been since I was about 17. We thought we were careful. I remember my period was late.[82]

> I got pregnant after a condom split AND I took the morning after pill within 24 hours. It was October 27th 2010 when I found out I was pregnant, in a disabled toilet so my BF [boyfriend]

could be with me while we read it, as doing the test at home was too risky for both of us. I was in 6th year and studying for my leaving.[83]

Moreover, violence and stealthing resulted in crisis pregnancies. Some people who contributed to *In Her Shoes* told stories of intimate-partner violence that precluded them from using birth control, and others described stealthing that led to pregnancies:

I had been seeing the guy for a little over 6 months, we always used condoms until I found out that he actually wasn't. He put a condom on and then midway through I found out that he had been taking it off.[84]

We only had sex 3 times, I took the pill, he used a condom. So he said. Later he confessed that he removed it once because he felt like "I could be the mother of his children." I still hate him for this.[85]

Irish women's reliance on less reliable forms of birth control is explained, in part, by cost—LARC methods can be expensive upfront—but also by popular misconceptions, a lack of information, and the limits of a medical system that to date has failed to train physicians adequately on LARC methods. An activist who spoke with us explained:

Take up of LARC has been very low in Ireland and that's because of the upfront costs involved, and also a real lack of information about them. You often hear from women that you need to have a baby before you can get LARC, it just hasn't been promoted really as an effective method.... Surveys show there's a relatively low take-up of contraception in Ireland because of access and the cost.

Intrauterine devices account for only 7.5% of birth control use in Irish women.[86] A 2014 survey demonstrated that Irish women did not know much about IUDs: 40% said that they could not say if the benefits of IUDs outweighed the risks, and only 57% of those surveyed understood what an IUD was.[87] A Galway-based university student interviewed in 2014 about LARC methods related, "Just . . . well me and my friends we, like, don't know what they are, don't know how many other things are out there . . . how good are they are compared to the pill or are they the same." Another student identified cost as a barrier to LARC use:

> Well like ideally I would love to be able to like fork out like two hundred euro to have like the implant or something, but as a student like I can't really afford that, so I suppose [the birth control pill is] just like the easiest form for me to take.[88]

Irish healthcare practitioners, as mentioned, also contribute to a lack of LARC uptake. A 2014 study found that physicians were most familiar with the birth control pill and most comfortable prescribing it, as opposed to LARC methods, to women. Conversations between physicians and women about LARC were rare. One physician in the 2014 study told researchers:

> I think the majority [of patients] still express a preference for the oral contraceptive. It is the euphemism for contraception, oh it's definitely the pill would be the preference. . . . Oh there's no doubt about it. It's still probably I'd say 1 in 4 of them, that's all that would be looking for long-term thing, really, in the grand scale of things. In my practice, most just want the pill.[89]

Most studies also suggest that many women are only told about LARC methods after having at least one child, with some physicians implying that LARC methods are not viable until after a pregnancy.[90] One woman posted on social media:

> When I finally made the decision to go hormone-free and seek getting the coil while still living in Ireland I was point blank refused for the reasons of "you haven't had kids yet, you might want them very soon" "this type of contraception is slightly too long lasting for someone your age." The opinion in Ireland seems to be that even though I was having many problems with contraceptives containing hormones, my safest and most reasonable option of contraception was prematurely taken away from me because "I was in childbearing age."[91]

This may explain why in Ireland IUDs are more commonly prescribed to older women who already have children rather than younger women with no pregnancies.

These realities proved frustrating to the activists and advocates we interviewed. As one told us:

> All the international evidence suggests LARC is most effective so it's simple, and I, you know, easy peasy, that's what all the evidence suggests, that's the really frustrating thing, we're not the first country in the world to introduce a termination service, we're not the first country in the world to look at contraception, we need to learn from the evidence that's out there, and LARC is very clearly, you can put LARC in on the day of [pregnancy termination] and that's what we need to do, if you really genuinely want to minimize your number of terminations you need to address, actively address contraception.

Another activist agreed, remarking:

What we're saying is, if you look at the evidence and you want to keep the abortion rates low, you need to focus on contraception. One of my favorites is in Switzerland, they reformed the law in 2002, and the abortion rate came down because it included a provision for better access to contraception. The bit that was missing from that, is that it's not just contraception, it's the long-acting contraception, they're the ones that really reduce the impact of unintended pregnancy.

While most advocates we interviewed supported greater LARC uptake, the issue, from a reproductive justice standpoint, can be fraught. Although research in Ireland is scarce, work conducted on the United States demonstrates that LARC methods are often prescribed more often for low-income women, unmarried mothers, and women of color. Physicians and other healthcare providers, then, "continue to display individual bias based on patients' markers of difference . . . that impact their contraceptive recommendations." A long history of reproductive coercion and violence in the United States, including forced sterilization of women of color, has compromised some women's trust in long-acting methods.[92] Reproductive justice scholars caution that promoting the use of particular forms of contraception, particularly amongst marginalized communities, risks associations with coercion.[93] Pushing LARC methods, then, as well as withholding LARC methods and sterilization, can be harmful in some contexts and viewed as oppressive by some. While there is no definitive evidence of coercion of women of color in Ireland to date, the country's unique history again matters, perhaps complicating trust in the medical system and the patient-doctor relationship. The forced hysterectomy scandal and symphysiotomy, discussed in chapter 6, are both clear evidence of this. In addition, some evidence suggests that Traveller women are encouraged to seek LARC and/or sterilization at higher levels than settled women.[94]

CONCLUSION: MOVING FORWARD

In 2012, a government report stated:

> A significant investment has been made in sexual health protec-
> tion and crisis pregnancy activities over a ten-year period. . . . We
> have seen the initiation and implementation of highly effec-
> tive national social marketing campaigns designed to challenge
> behavioural and attitudinal norms that give rise to unsafe sexual
> behaviours.[95]

Still, evidence since 2012 suggests that ignorance and misinformation persist. There is much more to be done to address the historical, cultural, and structural barriers to contraceptive use in Ireland
today. Grassroots organizing and truth-telling that feature ordinary stories and embodied realities can help. In 2020, for example,
a #MyMorningAfter panel at University College Cork brought
together students and activists to talk about emergency contraception experiences. As the event's organizers remarked:

> The more you talk about it, the less shameful it is. You take the
> sting out of it and I think if you all get up and share mortifying
> stories of going to the chemist and buying the morning-after pill,
> it becomes a lot less mortifying. You're all in it together.[96]

Government efforts continue as well; the 2019 Report of the
Working Group on Contraception outlined a three-part strategy
under the Health Ireland Framework moving forward:

- Everyone in Ireland will receive comprehensive and age-
  appropriate sexual health education/information and will
  have access to appropriate prevention and promotion services;

- Equitable, accessible and high-quality sexual health services, which are targeted and tailored to need, will be available to everyone; and
- Robust and high-quality sexual health information will be generated to underpin policy, practice, service planning and strategic monitoring.[97]

By budgeting for free contraception in 2022, the government has taken essential, concrete steps to increase birth control access for all people in Ireland. Still, research on the experiences, stories, and viewpoints of women remain scarce. Reid and Taylor write that "the provision of maternity care continues to be governed by a medical industrialized model, which emphasizes the economic and administrative needs of hospitals rather than focusing on the needs of women."[98] Moving forward, approaching contraception—along with other aspects of women's health—from an intersectional and reproductive justice perspective can help increase access, knowledge, and truth-telling in the Republic of Ireland.

Abortion

Discussing the 2018 mobilization of Repeal advocates—those who came together to encourage Irish people to vote to overturn the divisive anti-abortion Eighth Amendment (1983)—one activist we interviewed recalled:

> So we talked about setting up some type of group and then, what happened was Youth Defense, which was pretty much funded by the US and US groups, did [an anti-abortion] campaign. . . . A bunch of us were really angry so we came together to see what we could do, to stop that. A day long workshop and organizing type of thing was held in the social center; out of that formed the Abortion Rights Network, I think it was called. So what eventually came out of that was the Abortion Rights Campaign, those people that were there and signed up to get involved in certain types of work whether it was media work, direct action, creative stuff, and that formed in a way the bones of a campaign.

Activists whom we spoke to, like this one, brought attention to the uniqueness of Ireland's abortion-rights campaign while placing it a comparative context. Several interviews highlighted the inspiration that Irish activists found in global feminist movements; others

Catching Fire. Beth Sundstrom and Cara Delay, Oxford University Press. © Oxford University Press 2023. DOI: 10.1093/oso/9780197743942.003.0004

described the involvement of American anti-choice organizations and money in attempting to influence an anti-abortion "no" vote in the 2018 referendum. The participant quoted here also articulated the methods of the Repeal movement: "media work, direct action, creative stuff," which were discussed even at initial meetings. In the months leading up to the May 2018 referendum, these methods, and in particular story-telling and truth-telling via digital media, helped convince ordinary citizens to vote to decriminalize abortion for the first time in the island's modern history. The referendum to repeal the Eighth Amendment succeeded, with over 65% of Ireland's voting public supporting it. In 2018, the Health (Regulation of Termination of Pregnancy) Act provided for abortion in the Republic of Ireland up to twelve weeks of pregnancy; the Act was implemented in early 2019.[1]

This chapter analyzes the legal and political contexts of abortion and abortion-rights activism in Ireland. It asks how and why the Repeal movement succeeded in 2018 and explores the historical origins of this movement and its transnational influences. Assessing the methods and messages that Repeal campaigners utilized, it demonstrates how a focus on truth-telling and personal narratives, publicized through various forms of digital media and art, helped to convince ordinary Irish people to vote "yes" in 2018. Since Repeal, numerous scholars have analyzed story-telling-as-strategy in Irish feminist activism.[2] This chapter is distinct in that it places an examination of methods alongside the *content* of the stories that women told and the voices that the campaign highlighted. It was not only how narratives were expressed, we argue, but also the themes they articulated, including bodily experiences and cross-generational support, that affected public opinion. This investigation also interrogates the stories that were told—and those that were not told—during and after Repeal. It asks how and why the voices of medical professionals were featured in the Together for Yes movement and how some voices—those of migrants, for example—were often obscured or ignored in the mainstream campaign.

The successful 2018 Repeal movement, the chapter posits, is linked to a particular moment: a "moment of post-shame storytelling"[3] in Ireland that found its expression in the thriving world of feminist digital activism and that told particular stories. This chapter also recognizes, like the activists we interviewed have, that this moment was a long time coming, following a decades-long movement for abortion rights and access. Our analysis also moves beyond 2018 to ask how activists have continued their work in a post-Repeal landscape, how they have reflected on the successes and limits of the Repeal movement within the framework of reproductive justice, and how they are addressing contemporary issues, including a current review of the Republic's 2019 abortion legislation as well as abortion access during the COVID-19 pandemic.

HISTORY, REPRODUCTIVE JUSTICE, AND ABORTION

An intersectional analysis of abortion-seeking women reminds us that not only gender but also class, race, sexuality, region, and a person's legal status impact access to abortion. Here, again, Ireland's twentieth-century postcolonial history matters; it affected and continues to affect abortion access. In February 2018, a contributor to *In Her Shoes*, a campaign on Twitter and Facebook that allowed people to anonymously share their abortion stories in the lead up to the May referendum on the Eighth Amendment, wrote:

> [Ireland is] a country bound to the laws of a religion that has failed many people in Ireland. A religion that has objectified women for so long, a religion that has ignored and covered up

child abuse stories within the catholic church, a religion that opposed homosexuality [and] equal marriage. The Church has been on the wrong side of history and women at every turn, and 2018 should be the year of complete change.[4]

As this person noted, in the weeks and months before the 2018 referendum, many people framed discussions of abortion in Ireland within the context of the country's past, and specifically the Church-state consensus that informed almost all aspects of legal and political life throughout much of the twentieth century. The state's religious ethos affected medical care; consequently, a Catholic-informed bio-medical model that was antithetical to women's bodily autonomy dominated healthcare.[5]

As chapter 2 demonstrated, upon independence in 1922, the Free State (and later Éire and the Republic of Ireland) sought to promote marital fertility and restrict access to fertility control. As part of this agenda, in addition to limiting access to and information about contraception, the new state retained Britain's 1861 anti-abortion Offences Against the Person Act, which read as follows:

Every woman, being with child, who, with intent to procure her own miscarriage, shall unlawfully administer to herself any poison or other noxious thing, or shall unlawfully use any instrument or other means whatsoever with the like intent; and whosoever, with intent to procure the miscarriage of any woman, whether she be or be not with child, shall unlawfully administer to her or cause to be taken by her any poison or other noxious thing, or shall unlawfully use any instrument or other means whatsoever with the like intent, shall be guilty of a felony, and being convicted thereof shall be liable . . . to be kept in penal servitude for life. . . . Whosoever shall unlawfully supply or procure any poison or other noxious thing, or any instrument or thing whatsoever, knowing that the same is intended to be unlawfully used or employed with intent to procure the miscarriage of any woman, whether she be or be not with child, shall be guilty of a misdemeanor, and being convicted thereof shall be liable . . . to be kept in penal servitude . . .[6]

Of course, criminality did not prevent abortions; the work of several historians has provided extensive evidence for a thriving clandestine criminal abortion industry throughout most of the twentieth century.[7] The general pattern of criminal abortion in Ireland before the 1970s involved abortions on Irish soil, sometimes at the hands of quasi-"professional" practitioners and sometimes with the assistance of friends and neighbors. While prosecutions for abortion-related offenses occurred, they were relatively uncommon, linked to those rare cases in which medical complications or even death followed criminal procedures. A few sensational cases, most notably the 1956 trial of former nurse-midwife Mamie Cadden, created a link in the popular mind between abortion, death, and criminality, which likely helped buoy anti-abortion attitudes throughout the rest of the century.[8] Cadden, one of several abortion providers working in Dublin in the 1940s and 1950s, was arrested on murder charges after the death of one of her clients. Convicted of murder and sentenced to death, Cadden later died in an insane asylum.[9] The vast majority of criminal abortions throughout the twentieth century, however, appear to have been successful and were not detected by authorities.[10]

After 1967, when most of the United Kingdom, except for Northern Ireland, legalized abortion, Irish women seem to have moved away from criminal abortions on Irish soil, instead accessing the "abortion trail" by traveling to the United Kingdom, and most commonly England, to receive legal procedures.[11] From 1970 to 2015, at least 180,000 women from the Republic embarked on the "trail," seeking abortions abroad.[12] The reality that thousands of Irish women had to leave home and cross national borders to access medical services has been problematized by feminist scholars and placed within the larger context of what Caelainn Hogan calls the "shame-industrial complex."[13] Scholars have also argued that the containment or exile of so-called "deviant" women was essential to maintaining the purity of the nation in the twentieth century. The success of the Irish nation in the twentieth century, as philosopher Clara Fischer writes, relied on "the physical excising of women's bodies, either in institutions or through effective removal to other jurisdictions for abortion access."[14]

Approaching abortion in Ireland through a reproductive justice framework encourages us to confront the real-world contexts, including travel, that women faced when trying to access services before 2019. Indeed, abortion travel during the era of criminality was a central topic discussed by both our interviewees and those who posted to social media sites such as *In Her Shoes* in 2018. These accounts emphasized the financial burdens of travel, feelings of isolation and alienation, and fear of being discovered. A woman involved in abortion counseling whom we interviewed, for example, said:

> But really what we found from our counseling services was the difficulty of travel. Being delayed, not getting appropriate services, traveling without good information. The impact of having to get the money together, documentation, migrant women and women who couldn't travel, we were barred from helping women financially with the costs and helping anyone who didn't get to travel, so they were coerced into being parents against their wishes.

In 2018, a contributor to *In Her Shoes* posted: "Travelling was the worst. I felt like I was looking over my shoulder all the time. Checking to see if I recognized anyone on the plane."[15] Another wrote:

The father of the baby told me it was my decision, but he wanted me to have an abortion. Even though the idea horrified me, I asked him how we could arrange this when neither of us had money and we'd have to travel to England and pay for flights, accommodation and a procedure. My parents would certainly notice their young daughter was missing for a few days. He told me he would find a way to get the money together to send me over. Send me, not join me. And he made it very clear that he would not support me, or the baby, if I continued with the pregnancy.[16]

Travel added to the stress of a crisis pregnancy by bringing additional traumas, including feelings of loneliness and isolation and the uncertainties of navigating unfamiliar spaces.

The secrecy and lies that abortion travel required increased burdens and compounded trauma.[17] Jean, who had an abortion in England in the 1990s, told researchers:

The practical arrangements seemed enormous. I would have to travel alone or we would have to invent a weekend away. That would involve endless lies to the children, family and friends. Going alone was by far the better option in one way, but it felt lonely and frightening to travel alone for an operation.[18]

Furthermore, the experience of travel served to complicate some women's relationships with their home nation. As Michaela Carroll and colleagues write: "The individual accounts featured on *In Her Shoes* consistently linked the personal with the national. The lies that women told in their own lives mirrored the greater lie that Irish society upheld for decades: the myth that Ireland, unlike other places, did not have 'vices' such as abortion."[19]

Even as abortion remained criminalized in Ireland under the 1861 Offences Against the Person Act and thousands of women continued to travel to the United Kingdom for terminations, the abortion landscape changed significantly in 1983 with the Eighth Amendment to the Irish Constitution. After a popular referendum in which over 60% of the population voted in favor of adopting this amendment, the Constitution was changed. The Eighth Amendment specified: "The State acknowledges the right to life of the unborn and, with due regard to the equal right to life of the mother, guarantees in its laws to respect, and, as far as practicable, by its laws to defend and vindicate that right."[20] The campaign in favor of the Eighth Amendment was born, in part, from developments that occurred outside of Ireland, notably the 1967 decriminalization of abortion in most of the United Kingdom and the 1973 *Roe v. Wade* decision in the United States. Some anti-abortion activists in Ireland feared that this abortion liberalization would be contagious, and "across the next few decades, attempts to protect Ireland and Irishness—defined as Catholic and conservative—from the moral bankruptcy of the modern world characterized national politics and culture."[21] Moreover, as Cara Delay writes, "The Catholic Church stepped directly into debates over the moral future of the island. Less than a decade after Pope Paul VI's *Humanae Vitae*, Irish Bishops warned in a 1975 publication *Human Life Is Sacred* that Ireland's traditional values were increasingly under siege and affirmed that her people must recognize and defend 'the absolute rights of unborn life.'"[22] The successful campaign to pass the Eighth Amendment in the early 1980s was an important moment in exposing the transnational nature of abortion debates and how Irish anti-abortion campaigners were influenced by external forces. As this chapter will discuss later, the 2018 anti-Repeal movement witnessed similar developments.

In the 1990s, 2000s, and 2010s, a series of scandals and legal challenges to the Eighth Amendment brought abortion to the Irish public's attention and mobilized abortion-rights activists, helping them develop the tactics that would ultimately lead to the amendment's repeal in 2018. First, what is known as the "X" case troubled Ireland's anti-abortion consensus in 1992. "X," a 14-year-old girl, had been raped by a family acquaintance, becoming pregnant. Her parents made plans to take "X" to Britain for an abortion, contacting the Irish police before they left to ask if they should bring back fetal tissue for DNA analysis that would help the state prosecute the rapist. In response, the Attorney General, citing the Eighth Amendment's wording on fetal rights, placed an injunction on "X," forbidding her from leaving the country and, thereby, preventing her from traveling to receive a legal abortion in Britain. After an appeal to the Supreme Court, "X" ultimately was allowed to travel for an abortion. Polls at the time demonstrated that most Irish people opposed legalizing abortion in Ireland but supported travel to Britain for abortion.[23] The "X" case ushered in an age of legal uncertainty in Ireland. In 1992, as a direct result of the "X" scandal, the Thirteenth and Fourteenth amendments to the Irish Constitution, approved by the public, allowed for abortion travel and the dissemination of information within Ireland about abortion services abroad but affirmed that abortion would still be criminalized on Irish soil.[24] The "X" case also brought international attention to Ireland's abortion restrictions; politicians from other European Union states, for example, expressed horror at the plight of "X" and Ireland's laws.[25]

The years 2009 and 2010 witnessed more tragic abortion-related cases with implications for the legal status of terminations in Ireland and Ireland's international status and reputation. First, a legal case, *A. B. and C. v. Ireland*, came before the European Court of Human Rights. Three women, identified only as "A," "B," and "C," brought the suit to the Court, claiming "that Ireland violated the Convention for the Protection of Human Rights and Fundamental Freedoms, 1950" by forcing them to travel to Britain for abortions.[26] Then, in

2010, Michelle Harte, a woman with a wanted pregnancy who was advised by doctors to terminate because she was also fighting cancer, was denied an abortion by a Cork hospital committee. She had to travel to Britain for the procedure; the delay in the procedure may have contributed to her subsequent death from cancer.[27]

The key turning point in attitudes to abortion, and a catalyst for both activism and legal reform, was the Savita Halappanavar case in 2012. Halappanavar died in October 2012 of sepsis after being refused a therapeutic and medically necessary abortion at a Galway hospital. Reports at the time claimed that nurses and doctors who were treating Halappanavar told her and her husband that they could not perform a necessary abortion because of Ireland's Catholic-informed laws and ethos. The outcry following Halappanavar's death led to abortion-rights marches and significant activist mobilization.[28] "Within days of the story becoming public," writes David Ralph, "an incensed crowd of upwards of 20,000 marched throughout the streets of Dublin and chanted, 'NEVER AGAIN, NEVER AGAIN, NEVER AGAIN.' "[29]

Here, again, an international outcry mobilized abortion-rights activists. British news outlets, including *Sky News*, led with Halappanavar's death the same day that the news broke in Ireland, and the *India Times* carried the headline "Ireland Murders Pregnant Indian Dentist."[30]

The Halappanavar case brought legal and constitutional changes. The 2013 Protection of Life During Pregnancy Act technically left room for a legal abortion in Ireland if a pregnant woman's life was at risk. However, legal confusion persisted, and few abortions were performed in Ireland. Over the next few years, legal cases also brought Ireland's violations of women's rights to international courts. The United Nations Human Rights Committee (UNHRC) considered several cases on abortion in Ireland in 2016. It found that Irish anti-abortion policies had violated women's rights, calling "on Ireland to introduce 'accessible procedures for pregnancy termination' to prevent similar violations in the future." As The *Guardian* reported at the time, "The judgment marks the first time that an international human rights committee has recognised that by criminalising abortion, a state has violated a woman's human rights."[31]

By 2016, the government was ready to put the issue of abortion to the Irish public. It commissioned a Citizens' Assembly to discuss the issue; its members met and debated over several weeks, ultimately voting that Ireland should consider legalizing abortion.[32] Early 2018 brought an announcement that the government had scheduled a popular referendum on repealing the Eighth Amendment for May 2018. As abortion-rights activists mobilized for the Repeal campaign, they aimed to showcase women's abortion narratives and experiences, focusing on truth-telling to humanize and normalize abortion.

TRUTH-TELLING

Truth-telling in terms of women's abortion experiences, which became a central method during the Repeal campaign of 2018, required an explicit, vocal rejection of the silences and secrecies of Irish history and culture; women who shared their narratives on social media often reflected on the silence, shame, and stigma that surrounded their pregnancy terminations in an age of abortion criminality. The Repeal movement in Ireland placed ordinary women's experiences and stories at the center of analysis and provided platforms for women to tell their truths anonymously and in their own words. By doing so, these movements attempted to overcome the shame, the fear, and especially, the silence that had long dominated Irish women's reproductive experiences, and particularly abortion. Women posting about their abortion experiences rejected the past and attempted to create a better future: one in which women's voices would be heard and taken seriously.

Since the successful referendum in 2018, many scholars have demonstrated how and why women's story-telling proved essential in the Repeal movement. "By talking about abortion," writes David Ralph, "openly, freely, genuinely—the stigma surrounding it will be reduced, the procedure normalised."[33] Abortion story-telling, as Katie Mishler writes, "serves as a powerful intervention into cultural and national narratives of gender, motherhood, and femininity, countering restrictive, essentialist ideologies with embodied experience."[34] In order to get these messages out before Repeal, feminist activists organized into several groups in the "Together for Yes" movement. Three organizations led this movement: the Abortion Rights Campaign, the National Women's Council of Ireland, and the Coalition to Repeal the Eighth Amendment. According to umbrella Together for Yes organization, "We represent those people who believe that Ireland is a compassionate country which needs laws that reflect the reality of people's lives. We represent those people who believe that we must support, respect and protect women in their time of greatest need."[35] The campaign focused on grassroots efforts and a robust social media presence and was determined, from its inception, to feature women's experiences.

It is also important to note that Repeal activists also explicitly called on the tactics of other campaigns as they honed their methods. Door-to-door canvassing was a strategy that borrowed from the history of feminist organizing but had also brought great success several years earlier during another movement: marriage equality. In the lead-up to a 2015 popular referendum on legalizing marriage for LGBTQ+ people, "Yes" campaigners realized that their best approach was a personal one, based on individuals' experiences and stories. They identified "the need to tap into the rich vein of personal stories that was already emerging online and offline, which, if communicated authentically to voters, might determine the outcome."[36]

In the marriage equality vote, personal stories had a clear effect; consequently, activists seeking to repeal the Eighth Amendment in 2018 adopted these story-telling tactics as well.[37]

Activist strategies during Repeal included a physical claiming of space through canvassing, protests, and marches, which were all adapted from earlier social justice movements, including first- and second-wave feminism. Advocates for reform also employed other strategies, such as activism through art. Rachael Young explores how street art, notably murals, served as a way for artivists to claim space and force a public reckoning of abortion. In her analysis of street artist Maser's Repeal mural in Dublin, Young argues that murals "created a forum-like space, both corporeal and virtual, and allowed Irish citizens to interact with feminist issues and debates in their daily lives."[38] Arts activism, with origins as far back as the 1990s, was central to publicizing and personalizing the Repeal movement. Street art, murals, graffiti, plays, poetry, music, public readings, and other performances—"embodied actions of feminists in place," in the words of Lorna O'Hara—claimed space in Ireland and abroad.[39] The Artists' Campaign to Repeal the Eighth Amendment, for example, was active across Ireland in the weeks before the referendum. In April 2018, it organized a procession in Limerick featuring powerful banners. Alice Maher, one of the artivists involved, later reflected:

> I truly felt that by moving through those streets we actually changed something, there was something in the air in the city on that day, everyone went quiet, the traffic stopped, it was total silence. Silence is very powerful. It's powerful to make beautiful things as well. People rallied when they saw us coming.[40]

These approaches promoted activists' visibility, engaged the Irish public through visual forms, and featured the experiences of ordinary women.

Many artivists and arts activism organizations both staged physical, in-person events and utilized digital space to advocate for abortion reform. Speaking of I.M.E.L.D.A., a group that focuses on "direct-action feminist performance," held protests in London aimed at visiting Irish politicians, "tied a giant pair of knickers around the gates of Leinster House (the Irish Parliament building)," and created #knickersforchoice on Facebook and Twitter.[41] The Maser mural claimed physical space in Dublin but also made a splash online as a digital image, photographed and shared widely across social media platforms.[42]

The methods of the Repeal movement were certainly significant, but so, too, were its messages, which made visible women's embodied and emotional experiences and encouraged a sense of community. Contributors to *In Her Shoes* wrote about not only their individual experiences but also the struggles of others; many claimed that they were encouraged to participate because they were inspired by a sense of cross-generational solidarity that was finally allowing Irish women to break the silences of the past and create a better future. The themes of silence and breaking silences, for example, were present in contributors across age ranges and with different abortion experiences separated sometimes by decades. In a post from April 20, 2018, for example, a woman wrote: "I was 26 when I had my abortion, I've never spoken about it to anyone and I am now 62!"[43] Another posted: "When I was considering writing to you, I realised that despite the relatively 'liberal' circles I moved in, in 15 years I have never had a conversation with another woman in Ireland who has [told me she] had an abortion."[44]

In March 2018, a contributor shared: "It is because of this page that I found my voice, I have been silent a year now since I had to make the hardest decision of my life and it is with other women I stand side by side, for having been brave enough to share their story."[45] Numerous contributors also linked their own experiences and voices with not only women in the past but also their future hopes for their daughters or granddaughters. One woman, describing her own abortion travel experience, revealed that her mother, who traveled with her, also had an abortion decades previously. The daughter's experience "brought up all the old feelings of shame" for the mother, but together they were able to work through those emotions and even strengthen their relationship.[46] Another contributor shared that her abortion experience inspired her mother to vote for Repeal:

> I'm so proud of my mam for recognizing that she's really pro-choice, and still knowing that she can be religious while supporting women and families in making the best decisions for themselves. She'll be voting to repeal the 8th. I think there's a lot of people of her generation that have stories to tell about the past, and want a better future for their daughters.[47]

These narratives generated cross-generational communication and support, which had long been difficult to maintain in an Ireland that prohibited such open discussions and, essentially, alienated women from each other through its culture of silence and secrecy.

Particularly noteworthy in abortion-rights activism was the role of social media. Through social media, Irish women made personal revelations, exercised their activist voices, and demanded national change. As one woman wrote on *In Her Shoes* on April 11, 2018, just a month before the referendum: "We will not and must not let our women down anymore. I am no longer your dirty secret, I am a woman of Ireland and you will hear me and you will listen."[48] While social media is often thought to be the platform of the young, many middle-aged Irish women used *In Her Shoes* to tell their abortion narratives for the first time. A June 2018 entry posted by an Irish woman who experienced a clandestine abortion decades earlier read as follows: "I have a 19 year old daughter now. I will be voting Yes for her and her generation. That she has a choice. That she won't have the hardship that I had. That she won't have to travel like I did, it's a hard decision made worse with having to go."[49]

Social media, in some cases, facilitated the telling of polyvocal stories. "To embrace the vision of reproductive justice," argue reproductive justice scholars Loretta Ross and Rickie Solinger, "one must embrace polyvocality—many voices telling their stories that together may be woven into a unified movement for human rights."[50] Hyesun Hwang and Kee-Ok Kim argue that

> social media [platforms] take the role of mediating users' interaction as a method of engaging and empowering people. Contrary to the traditional mobilization that combines individuals' resources to establish collective power through social movement organizations, the diverse voices can be effectively collectivized and transmitted to the society on social media.[51]

In the Irish abortion-rights activist campaign, story-telling and truth-telling via social media were empowering for some but also oppressive in other cases. Some who posted their stories on social media, for example, faced public backlash or trolling. In 2016, the Twitter handle @twowomentravel featured one Irish woman, accompanied by a friend, who shared her experiences traveling to England to access an abortion. "The Twitter feed bio, which read 'Two women, one procedure, 48 hours away from home," argue Claire Bracken and Cara Delay, "was an act of protest and solidarity (the feed started with a direct tweet to taoiseach Enda Kenny)."[52] Several Twitter users responded to this initiative, however, "with the hashtags #KeepLegsClosed and #ChoiceIsMurder; a Catholic blogger accused the two women of exploiting 'the destruction of human life for entertainment purposes.'"[53] Therefore, as Katherine Side reminds us, in some cases story-telling through social media resulted in further harms, with "historical patterns of shaming continu[ing] to be perpetuated."[54]

Abortion-rights advocates and activists confronted opposition to their views and social media presence within Ireland, of course, but also internationally. In fact, a group of US-based anti-abortion social media users targeted the *In Her Shoes* Facebook page in April 2018. They flooded the page with spam and posted "more than 200 one- and two-star reviews" to it. In response, the organizers of *In Her Shoes* posted:

> We would like to issue an apology to those that have been temporarily locked out of their account following attempts from pro-life organisations to silence women from sharing their lived experiences. Yesterday, pro-life accounts had been spamming and trolling numerous conversations within the *In Her Shoes* community. It is our duty to protect the people that are central to this conversation—women that have been negatively impacted by the 8th amendment.[55]

Together for Yes and other activist groups developed clear strategies to deal with trollers—as one activist told us, "we took a deliberate policy not to engage . . . just really not engage with the bots or trolls." Most decided that avoiding and ignoring anti-abortion forces was the best way forward.

It also became apparent in 2018, however, that online trolls had the potential to disrupt the social media platforms that were so essential to the Repeal movement. Here, again, activists mobilized. Some created Repeal Shield, a troll-blocking tool that protected sites like *In Her Shoes*. Repeal Shield organizers claimed that during just a few months in 2018, they blocked 16,000 trolls and harassers. One of the creators of Repeal Shield later said of their efforts:

Six people, none of whom had ever met, decided to [do] something about the foul online abuse from Anti-Choicers: the name calling, grotesque photos, misinformation, harassment. They set up a block tool whereby, when you subscribed to the free service, anybody blocked by the Shield was automatically blocked for you: "Blocking Trolls so you don't have to!"[56]

In addition, Facebook, just a few weeks before the scheduled referendum, banned advertisements on the referendum that were created outside of Ireland.[57] Abortion-rights activists, then, responded immediately and effectively to online bullying and trolling.

Of the 16,000 trolls that Repeal Shield blocked, almost 60% of were from North America; indeed, international anti-choice groups "saw the island, with just 4.7 million people, as the front line of a wider ideological battleground. In particular, right-wing anti-abortion groups in the United States were keen to maintain what they saw as one of the last bastions against abortion."[58] The healthcare and feminist activists whom we interviewed clearly recognized the American influence on the so-called "pro-life" campaign in Ireland. One told us: "We have clearly seen an attempt to import tactics from the US in US pro-life movements I mean that is clear—someone is also coaching these people." Another agreed that US influence was direct, remarking: "But some of the things [Irish 'pro-lifers'] were suggesting like compulsory ultrasounds and vaginal ultrasounds were as somebody said, straight out of the US playbook, so it seems to me that they are getting instructed." Some activists saw American influence in popular media campaigns as well:

> One example that really stuck with me, was a very kind of gendered newspaper advertisement which was directed at men and it said "Men Protect Life" and it was illustrated with a fireman carrying like three children out of a burning building, and the

fireman's uniform was an American uniform. So firemen in Ireland wear black jackets, and the fireman in this picture was wearing that kind of almost khaki green, with the reflective strips, kind of thing, which you just don't get in Ireland.

Irish abortion-rights advocates recognized not only how and why American anti-choice groups influenced or intervened in the Repeal debates but also the global and transnational influences and implications of their own movement. Some of our interviewees, for example, told us how inspired they were, after living abroad in places such as the United Kingdom and the United States, to share global feminist organizing and tactics with their Irish counterparts. Furthermore, since Repeal in 2018, the global implications of the Irish case have become evident. In October 2020, Poland implemented a near-total ban on abortion (similar to the pre-2018 situation in Ireland); a year later, a woman named Izabel died of sepsis after being denied a therapeutic abortion. The similarities between Izabel's case and that of Savita Halappanavar made the news, with some journalists and activists positing that Izabel's tragedy might help change Polish laws, like Halappanavar's did for Ireland.[59]

ABORTION ACTIVISM: WHOSE VOICES?

While some scholars have framed the Repeal movement as a new form of feminist activism in Ireland, the Repeal campaign built not only on other contemporary activist campaigns but also on a potent, yet still understudied, history of women's feminist activism in Ireland. Indeed, activists we spoke with consistently underscored the need to recognize the history of their movement, positioning the Eighth Amendment as a catalyst for it. "So I suppose [Repeal] happened," one told us, "because of activists' pressures over a number of years. If you look at the 1983 campaign and you look at the people that stayed involved afterwards, they really kept the grassroots." Katherine Side posits: "Advocacy for reform persisted for thirty-six years prior to Ireland's 2018 referendum on abortion, undertaken by individuals and groups who opposed the 1983 insertion of the Eighth Amendment in Bunreacht na hÉireann, the Irish Constitution."[60] Feminist and legal scholars have called attention to the decades-long work of advocates to enact gradual reforms in the Irish constitutional and legal systems. Speaking of the successful Repeal referendum in 2018, Joanne Conaghan argues:

> At the same time, we should not be dazzled by these most visible of achievements for they stand upon a foundation of equality-seeking reforms which, over the last 25 years, have slowly and steadily ratcheted up the momentum for change: let us not forget that homosexual acts were decriminalised in Ireland in 1993, that the constitutional prohibition on divorce was removed in 1996, or that, from the late 1990s, anti-discrimination laws were extended to protect gays, lesbians, and other socially disadvantaged groups.[61]

Historians' understandable focus on the oppressive patriarchal structures of twentieth-century Ireland have, at times, overshadowed the significant grassroots feminist movements that also characterized the age. Recent work has begun to uncover the importance of feminist activism in Irish history, highlighting the subversive tactics women used to circumvent silence and organize.[62] As Laura Kelly writes in her work on activists campaigning for contraceptive access, "the role of informal women's networks and the transmission of information between women that occurred outside the law were effective."[63] Irish women had a long history and tradition of organizing, one that was a necessary precursor to the Repeal movement.

Recognizing that the abortion-rights movement, as broad and diverse as it was, featured some voices while perhaps obscuring others is also significant. While Together for Yes and other abortion-rights groups insisted on the importance of the ordinary or everyday abortion story, they also gave significant time to particular voices, such as those of doctors and midwives. When Dr. Rhona Mahony, master of the National Maternity Hospital, Dublin, joined Together for Yes, different media outlets sought out her voice and views. Mahony, for example, along with another National Maternity Hospital physician, Dr. Peter Boylan, appeared in a video for Together for Yes. Featuring the voices of doctors, nurses, and midwives working within the existing healthcare system was a deliberate strategy. As a Repeal activist told us:

> What we did then, we realized that process and the medical voices were more critical to the debate than we had previously realized. They were seen by the general public as ... the so-called middle ground of the Irish Republic. We started to look at strategies to engage them, we looked at how we might open spaces or create safe spaces for them to talk about the issue and Irish abortion laws. We spent a lot of time with medical voices giving them space to talk through the issues, what would be an acceptable resolution from a healthcare position. The maternity hospitals, leading obstetricians and gynecologists in the country had the opportunity to talk amongst themselves and really discuss the issues. ... I think that had a huge impact, I think when we came to the referendum campaign it was pretty easy to make the decision that the debate should be focused on healthcare. That campaign could have been fought on moral, religious, human rights grounds, but I think the way it unfolded for most people were the medical voices and the voices of women who had abortions, had experienced the hands of traveling to another country.

As this narrative reveals, the experiences of those who traveled for abortion services before 2018 also were featured in mainstream abortion-rights campaigns. But while travel was, in fact, the experience of most abortion-seekers, some chose a different path: ordering abortion pills online and consuming them at home. The numbers of women who induced miscarriage through pills is unknown, but in 2014, Irish customs seized more than sixty packages containing abortion pills.[64] The stories of these women remained somewhat obscure in the mainstream Together for Yes movement. Also not emphasized as much as travel to the United Kingdom were the Irish women who utilized services provided by the Dutch group Women on Waves. In 2001, Women on Waves docked a ship off of the coast of Dublin (in international waters, so it would not be subject to Irish law) and gave abortions to Irish women there.[65]

Other voices that the abortion-rights movement emphasized included people who needed abortions because of a fatal fetal abnormality. Narratives of these experiences were viewed as perhaps more palatable to undecided or skeptical voters because they exposed that women with wanted pregnancies often needed abortions but had to travel to Britain for them. However, as Aideen O'Shaughnessy argues, the focus on these exceptional narratives and, overall, on "abortion as a negative affective object, one that is inherently connected to suffering and crisis," is problematic, helping to bolster the divide between "good" and "bad" abortions and impede the goal of normalizing all abortions.[66] One Repeal activist later recalled, "We had to push the 'good abortion and bad abortion' idea so it's a good abortion if there's a fatal fetal abnormality or you're dying but it's a bad abortion if like you just had an abortion because it was the right decision for you, we didn't do any of that." The activist group Termination for Medical Reasons (TFMR), furthermore, was deeply involved in Repeal activism. An activist told us:

And you know what's really shocking about it is that the very
first trope to come out and use personal stories to campaign for
abortion rights were the families who had been affected by fatal
fetal anomaly, termination for medical reasons. TFMR. This
really incredible group of very very dedicated family, women,
husbands, who were campaigning and the idea that someone in
that situation had been refused under the new legislation was
shocking to everyone.

While many Repeal activists recognized the need to tell the stories of
people facing fatal fetal abnormality, some would later question the
emphasis on these stories, which centered the rarer cases rather than
foregrounding the experiences of the majority of abortion-seekers.

Indeed, during and since the 2018 referendum, some of the limits
of the Repeal campaign have been criticized. Together for Yes, for
example, "received criticism for not engaging adequately with reproductive justice thinking and, particularly, with questions of race."[67]
The exclusion of migrant, refugee, and asylum-seeking women
from the mainstream campaigns was particularly troubling to some.
A focus on travel experiences, as Katie Mishler reminds us, "silences
the experiences of women who were not able to freely avail of medical tourism—disproportionately migrant women and particularly
those seeking asylum and living in direct provision."[68] Some of our
interviewees recognized these limitations and demonstrated their
awareness of the necessity of an intersectional approach to abortion
rights and access:

I think there was a cognizance on the ground among activists of
abortion being a class issue as well and that for so long, people
had this idea of middle-class women being able to afford to travel
to England to take care of things themselves, whereas that's not
an option for people from other backgrounds, to have the time,

money, resources to do those things. I suppose in that way it was very much cognizance of abortion being a class issue as well. Of course for like migrants, refugees, asylum seekers, there's a whole level of difficulty for them if they were to fall pregnant or were in need of a termination so I think there was very much a cognizance of the effects on different people from different backgrounds.

Still, the dominant image of the abortion-seeking woman continues, erroneously, to be a white, young, unmarried woman. Migrants and asylum-seekers, indeed, expressed that they felt left out during the Repeal movement. As one posted on the Migrants and Ethnic-minorities for Reproductive Justice (MERJ) website:

> So if you ask me what it's like to be a migrant woman in Ireland, coming from a country where abortion is legal I would describe it as a constant pressure. The pressure of knowing that your sexuality is covered in shame, that your reproductive health is criminalised. That your health depends on paperwork, money and, ultimately, privilege. A privilege you may not have. It is knowing that if you needed an abortion, you'd have to leave the country like a criminal, or you'd have to bow down and beg the authorities to let you do the best thing for you. It is also knowing that a different reality exists and that this is not normal.[69]

Other criticisms detailed the Repeal movement's focus on "women" rather than "pregnant people," which has been interpreted as dismissive of the rights of transgender people. One healthcare activist told us that the Together for Yes campaign deliberately did not foreground the experiences and needs of trans people because some in the movement believed it would alienate the Irish public:

So [we] were told "don't be foregrounding the fact that this is a trans issue in your press releases and stuff" so what we were doing was just putting in women and pregnant people and nobody cared, everyone's fine with it, but I remember very early on, there was this guy and he was an ex-Fianna Fáil, the most conservative party, so he was an ex-Fianna Fáil strategist who came to give us advice and my God did I learn about pure evil of how you canvas and how you influence people, he was very specific, he said "don't ever mention transpeople, don't even mention it, the people of Ireland will eat your face off" and when I was doing the Catholics for Choice training and I was doing a fake press conference and I was starting to talk about transpeople she said "Don't talk about trans" you would switch the focus, the journalist would be like "what do you mean, 'pregnant people'"?

As a result, the mainstream movement left some Irish people experiencing alienation rather than a sense of community, an issue that has become increasingly evident in the post-Repeal landscape. Recalls MERJ member Waszak:

During the campaign, we were always seen as an afterthought or some kind of niche issue, when the reality was that migrants and ethnic minorities were disproportionately affected by the 8th amendment, so best placed to be speaking about it and organising against it. And we know what happened and we remember who said what. But in hindsight after Repeal, some people wanted to just celebrate and move on. Some people did not want to remember the ugliness that they participated in, just the hero narrative that they brought abortion to Ireland in the end.[70]

CONCLUSION

In the wake of the 2018 referendum that repealed the Eighth Amendment, efforts to implement a legal system of abortion on the island for the first time in modern history began. As activist Ailbhe Smyth remarked, "I mean, the day after the referendum was the day that we started to have to do the hard work of making sure that women could actually access abortion in this country."[71] The new law—the Health (Regulation of Termination of Pregnancy) Act of 2018 (implemented in early 2019)—provides for abortion for any reason through twelve weeks of a pregnancy, but people seeking abortion must consult with at least two physicians and endure a three-day waiting period before their procedure. Interviewed several months after the referendum but before the new legislation was passed, an activist expressed concerns about some of the limitations of the proposed legislation:

> There's a lot of loopholes doctors can use that can put up barriers for women, if there's conscientious objection in legislation it needs to be down to fucking brass tacks, how specific, like how many hours a doctor needs to wait before he can pick up the phone and refer a woman to another doctor, how far can that doctor be, how long is she going to wait for that doctor, and so on. The time period in particular needs to be ... we call it refusal of care because it's more accurate than conscientious objection, but it needs to go on record immediately after he makes the call, that he refused care, so when there's the three year review, we can look back and see what's the profile of care refusal and see what we can do about that.

As this interviewee articulated, the 2018 legislation is problematic because it places obstacles in the way of women's access to care, and it also, significantly, perpetuates the historical trend of medicalizing reproduction and placing power in the hands of physicians.

Activist and advocacy group MERJ points out that the abortion system is deeply problematic in other ways. A required seventy-two-hour waiting period, the "conscientious objection" clause (the ability of practitioners to refuse to perform abortions), and the cost of abortion, according to MERJ, have effectively restricted access to abortion in general and for certain marginalized communities in particular, including migrants and asylum-seekers.[72] The shortfalls in the current system have ensured that the work of abortion-rights and reproductive justice activists and organizations, including MERJ, continues. Indeed, those we interviewed recognized the need to continue the momentum and persist with activism and advocacy:

> I suppose there's been a natural lull after the campaign which I think every group that did a lot of work on really felt, where you felt that you had a moment to breathe out of relief and just relax for a little while, but now I think this has kicked us back into gear, there's definitely much more to be achieved. Ireland simply doesn't have enough choice for women who are giving birth.

When it began in 2020, the COVID-19 epidemic also presented particular challenges for abortion access. Because access to abortion in Ireland is still limited—only ten of nineteen hospitals currently perform the procedure—many people continue to travel to the United Kingdom for termination services. The fact that abortion in Ireland is only legal for up to twelve weeks in a pregnancy means that women who need abortions after that time frame, many whose fetuses have fatal fetal abnormalities, also must travel. In fact, in 2020, 194 Irish women received abortions in the United Kingdom.[73] However, some who live in Ireland—notably asylum-seekers—are not permitted to leave the state until their legal status is settled; therefore, travel to Britain remains impossible for them.

During the COVID-19 pandemic, when in-person abortion consultations and surgical procedures were limited in some parts of the country, abortion access also was limited. The Irish Family Planning Association (IFPA) immediately encouraged the government to allow physicians to pivot to telemedicine and early medical abortion via the medications mifepristone and misoprostol.[74] These "abortion pills," as they are known, are proven to be both safe and effective and, thanks to services like Women on Web, have been used by Irish women, albeit illegally, for decades. In March 2020, "the Minister for Health told Dáil Eireann . . . that remote consultation for abortion care could be permitted without legislative amendment," paving the way for appointments via phone or videoconferencing and effectively allowing physicians to prescribe abortion pills that women can consume in their own homes.[75]

This development has brought an important question to light: should Irish women be able to access abortion pills via telemedicine even when the pandemic ends? Alison Spillane and colleagues argue that

> maintaining remote consultation as an option within the abortion care pathway could potentially improve access for a range of individuals, such as those living in rural areas, disabled people, and people with care responsibilities for whom in-person appointments may be logistically challenging. It would give patients more choice in service delivery modality, enabling them to access care in a manner consistent with their needs and preferences.[76]

Questions such as this are particularly timely given that the government's required three-year review of the Health (Regulation of

Termination of Pregnancy) Act occurred in 2022 and is, at the time of this writing (early 2023), pending release. The review was designed to "assess the operation and effectiveness of the law that came into force in January 2019, with consultation from service users, stakeholders and the public."[77]

As the state review of Ireland's abortion legislation continues, so do attempts to analyze the referendum and the Repeal movement as well as to document women's experiences of abortion in Ireland, past and present. These analyses have recognized the limits of the Together for Yes campaign while also pointing out how the larger methods of the Repeal movement, especially social media, allowed for broad, diverse, and intersectional feminist activism. Activists and scholars have published a plethora of books and articles since 2018, and in 2021, a coalition of archivists, scholars, and activists created a new project, Archiving the 8th. Funded in part by the Wellcome Trust and housed at University College Dublin, the project aims to "archive, collect, and research issues concerning women's reproductive health and rights, spanning the two abortion referenda in Ireland (1983–2018)." The group website calls for donations of "organisational records, political ephemera, websites/digital material and visual/material culture."[78] Archiving the 8th also has emphasized the importance of including narratives and experiences of marginalized peoples, demonstrating a keen awareness of the limitations of Repeal. It also promotes research and preservation as well as networking, encouraging researchers, for example, to conduct oral histories. Its archival project is extensive and inclusive, focusing on collecting not only physical artifacts or manuscripts but also digital movements, such as *In Her Shoes*. Therefore, Archiving the 8th hopes to document the stories of activists but is itself an activist movement, demonstrating the energy and vibrancy of feminist campaigners in a post-Repeal landscape.

Pregnancy

In July 2021, thousands of women's health activists in Dublin rallied against Church ownership of the new National Maternity Hospital with the same slogan—"Keep your rosaries away from my ovaries"— that feminists chanted thirty-eight years earlier to protest the creation of the Eighth Amendment in 1983.[1] Advocates carried signs stating "My womb is a secular state," "Nun of your business," and "Make our National Maternity Hospital public and secular."[2] The Campaign Against Church Ownership of Women's Healthcare organized the rally outside Leinster House because of continuing concerns that the new National Maternity Hospital, colloquially known as "the Baby Factory," would be built at the St. Vincent's University Hospital site in Elm Park, Dublin. Although the process to finalize the legal arrangements for the new hospital has been ongoing since 2013, the latest proposal involves the Religious Sisters of Charity order, who owns the land, leasing it to the state for 299 years.[3] The current proposal also includes equal representation on the Board of the Hospital for St. Vincent's, National Maternity Hospital directors, and the public interest.

Activists fear that giving not only ownership but also potentially decision-making powers to representatives of Ireland's Catholic Church will create further healthcare harms to women, potentially restricting access to essential services, such as contraception and

Catching Fire. Beth Sundstrom and Cara Delay, Oxford University Press. © Oxford University Press 2023. DOI: 10.1093/oso/9780197743942.003.0005

abortion. According to Peter Boylan, Minister for Health, "There isn't a single example in the entire world of a catholic institution owning land and allowing a maternity hospital to perform proce-dures which are directly contradictory to catholic teachings, such as sterilization and abortion."[4] A midwife we interviewed shared her concerns with us: "I think it's evil to think they're going to be refus-ing services . . . There needs to be a separation, and to say that there doesn't, and to say there's no impact is basically to just deny every single thing that's happened in Ireland. It's just insane to say it won't have an impact." Although protests about the National Maternity Hospital seem to reflect a lack of progress, one scholar and activist nuanced this theory, telling us, "I think people mobilized around that very quickly and it showed how much opposition there is to religious orders being involved in the care of pregnant women." Once again, women's health advocates identified the healthcare system as a site of Church and state regulation of women's reproduction in Ireland and led campaigns to oppose religious influence on maternity services.

This chapter will explicate Church and state involvement in wom-en's reproduction and deconstruct issues of identity and power by examining how medicalization has impacted the embodied experi-ence of pregnancy in Ireland. This chapter offers historical context to understand how pregnant women have made meaning of their bod-ies in the past and how that has changed. Through an analysis of the National Maternity Strategy and current maternity practices, it also explores how calls for woman-centered care intersect with practices of midwifery and the biomedical obstetric paradigm. Finally, an analysis of the *In Our Shoes—Covid Pregnancy* social media campaign, which shared anonymous narratives from women impacted by COVID-19 restrictions in Ireland, highlights the current context of debates on pregnancy rights, particularly the messages and campaigns involved in contemporary reproductive justice activism. Specifically, COVID-19 restrictions on maternity care may be understood as part of a long history of the Irish Church-state's control of women, and they exemplify the continued need for women to raise their voices through *In Our Shoes* to demand systemic change to ensure every woman's human right to high-quality, respectful maternity care.

WOMAN-CENTERED CARE

While Ireland today has a highly medicalized maternity system steeped in physician authority and biomedical power, these are relatively recent developments. When activists and healthcare professionals today talk about implementing a maternity model based on woman-centered care, they are, in some ways, advocating a return to the realities of the not-so-distant past. Lay Irish women were the main assistants at childbirth well into the twentieth century in many parts of Ireland, and most women, in both urban and rural parts of the island, continued to give birth at home until the 1940s or 1950s.[5] Home-based labor and birth were occasions dominated by women; often present at birth would be a laboring woman's female family members, other local women, and a handywoman—a lay midwife who gained her birthing wisdom from "a combination of personal experience, observation and intuition."[6] A woman whose mother was a handywoman from 1900 to 1920 later recalled:

> She was always ready to walk miles to deliver a baby, perhaps at
> night even, when a man could call for her, complete with his lan-
> tern, and they would set off over the hills and fields. I am well
> aware of the mothers and babies whose lives she saved.[7]

Men were rare in birthing rooms until hospitalization.

By the late nineteenth and early twentieth centuries, however, change was afoot: under the British colonial system, attempts to modernize and civilize Irish medical care resulted in formal training programs for nurses and midwives who assisted laboring and birthing women in homes.[8] These professional women, often outsiders in communities, brought a middle-class, reforming ethos to Irish homes, but they also sometimes worked together with handywomen and local women, keeping birth practices local and feminized. Doctors appeared in domestic births only rarely, and then only when complications occurred.[9] The process of medicalization, however, had begun, and it would accelerate rapidly in Ireland after independence. By the 1940s and 1950s, birth moved to hospitals where, as chapter 6 discusses, physician control of childbirth led to harmful practices, such as symphysiotomies.

In Ireland today, pregnancy is the number-one reason for admission to a hospital. Most women receive maternity services through hospitals, and 99% of women give birth in a hospital.[10] In fact, over one-third of all women give birth in one of three urban maternity hospitals in Dublin, including the Rotunda Hospital, The Coombe Women & Infants University Hospital, and the National Maternity Hospital.[11] Maternity care is predominately consultant or physician led, with service provided in a hospital. A midwife we interviewed described maternity care in Ireland: "It's a managed system of birth, it's an obstetric model of care." In some areas, DOMINO (Domiciliary In and Out) care is provided by a team of hospital-based community midwives through pregnancy, birth, and the postpartum period. In these cases, antenatal appointments may occur in the community or hospital. Women typically transfer home twelve to twenty-four hours after hospital-based childbirth, with midwives providing postnatal care at home. DOMINO is limited to certain geographic locations, and in 2014, it accounted for approximately 3.35% of total births in Ireland.[12] A large proportion of women choose combined care provided by the Maternity and Infant Care Scheme, which includes services shared between a general practitioner and the hospital/

DOMINO for antenatal, labor and delivery, and postnatal visits. For most women, postnatal care is provided by public health nurses at home. Low-risk women in certain geographic locations, such as Drogheda and Cavan, may choose midwife-led units co-located with a consultant-led unit. In this case, antenatal, intrapartum, and postnatal care are delivered by midwives in the community and in an alongside midwife-led unit, which is close to a traditional labor ward in case of emergency. This approach accounted for only approximately 0.6% of all births in Ireland in 2014,[13] despite the fact that it is clearly beneficial: a recent study found that midwifery-led antenatal care was associated with significantly higher rates of normal delivery.[14]

The Health Service Executive (HSE) also covers the cost of home births through a small number of self-employed community midwives, who provide care throughout pregnancy, childbirth, and postnatally. In 2014, home births accounted for approximately 0.2% of births in Ireland.[15] Unfortunately, home births are only available to low-risk women and those who live in certain geographic areas, based on midwife availability. A midwife we interviewed described the challenges of homebirths in Ireland:

> You can't just decide to have a homebirth you have to be signed off by a consultant that you're eligible for a homebirth so it's not just something a woman can decide to do by herself. [She has to] have a doctor say 'you're deemed suitable for this' and obviously then, if she's deemed slightly overweight, if she has any kind of myriad of health problems, previously which don't cause trouble, if she doesn't live in the right area . . . If there's any kind of problem in her pregnancy she can be immediately referred back to hospital care.

In the wake of Savita Halappanavar's 2012 death, the Irish Health Information and Quality Authority (HIQA) published an

*Investigation into The Safety, Quality and Standards of SERVICES
PROVIDED by the Health Service Executive to Patients, Including
Pregnant Women, at Risk of Clinical Deterioration, Including Those
Provided in University Hospital Galway, and as Reflected in the Care and
Treatment Provided to Savita Halappanavar.*[16] Ultimately, the report
recommended the development of a strategy to deliver a standard, consistent national maternity service model. In 2016, HIQA
released the first *National Standards for Safer Better Maternity Services*,
and the Minister for Health launched a *Creating a Better Future
Together: National Maternity Strategy 2016–2026.*[17] A women's health
activist described the need for the new maternity strategy:

> The impetus behind that was unfortunately high maternal death,
> poor birth outcomes, and there was an emphasis that it needed
> to be about women's decision making and women's choices in
> maternity care had to be brought to the fore much more . . . we
> also would have member groups work with women in maternity
> services and they're all about putting women's voices in the cen-
> ter of that kind of care. So in a lot of countries women have no
> say in the kind of birth method they're going to have and I think
> there's been an understanding that maternity care, because of the
> 8th amendment and because of the religiosity of Ireland that the
> emphasis has been on the child and not so much the woman.

Developing a national maternity strategy illustrated the urgency of
elevating women's health issues in the national discourse and developing a plan to address failures in the current system.

According to HIQA, the maternity strategy includes significant restructuring and reform of maternity and neonatal services,
including improved access and choice for women through maternity
networks and enhanced care pathways.[18] The National Maternity
Strategy outlines one model of care with three separate care pathways.

The Chair of the Maternity Strategy Steering Group acknowledged that childbirth is a "natural, physiological process" and that maternity services "should support the normalization of pregnancy and birth and women should be encouraged, and supported, to make their individual experience as positive as possible."[19] Although the report suggests that women should be offered choice regarding their preferred pathway of care, available choices are dictated by perceived clinical needs and ambiguous "best practices." Specifically, choice of pathway is determined by risk profile, including normal risk, medium risk, or high risk. The *Supported Care* pathway is intended for normal-risk mothers, with midwives leading care. The *Assisted Care* pathway is intended for medium-risk mothers, with care delivered by obstetricians and midwives. The *Specialized Care* pathway is intended for high-risk mothers and led by an obstetrician. Women in the *Supported Care* pathway may choose a homebirth or give birth in an alongside birth center, in close proximity to a traditional labor ward. Women in the *Assisted Care* or *Specialized Care* pathways give birth in a current labor ward, identified as a specialized birth center.

The National Maternity Strategy identifies a vision for maternity services in Ireland: "Women and babies have access to safe, high quality care in a setting that is most appropriate to their needs; women and families are placed at the centre of all services, and are treated with dignity, respect and compassion; parents are supported before, during and after pregnancy to allow them to give their child the best possible start in life."[20] A number of strategic priorities were identified to help realize this vision, including a focus on woman-centered maternity care. One of these priorities includes that "pregnancy and birth is recognized as a normal physiological process, and insofar as it is safe to do so, a woman's choice is facilitated." Although the strategy aims to center women, it is clear that a woman's choice will only be facilitated when it is deemed "safe to do so" by a health-care provider.

The reality that a healthcare provider will determine whether or not a woman's choice is "safe" is particularly problematic in the context of the history of the Eighth Amendment. Through the 2018 campaign to repeal the Eighth Amendment, many women's health activists realized that individuals in Ireland didn't know women couldn't refuse consent to treatment during pregnancy and childbirth. As one women's health professional we interviewed explained, "There was an asterisk that [informed consent] did not apply to pregnant women because of the 8th amendment. There was this well worked consent policy that didn't apply to one group only and that was pregnant women." Another activist shared:

> There were really big impacts around the autonomy of mothers and child birthing in Ireland, and we know now that the consent guidelines do not apply to the case of pregnant women, so there were a lot of big impacts there and the reality is most of the health services in Ireland have been religious ones and that has impacted so many services . . . that a moralistic approach to sexuality has been very clear for women.

A recent participatory action research study found that women's experiences of informed choice were dependent on the quality of their relationship with carers and their ability to engage in shared decision-making.[21] Lack of autonomy and lack of participation in decision-making during pregnancy and childbirth diminished women's sense of self.[22] Midwifery-led care alone resulted in a reciprocal relationship, which empowered women and inspired a sense of confidence.[23]

The National Maternity Strategy emphasizes that the service should be woman-centered, while acknowledging the important role of the partner and family. Indeed, the strategy supports a partnership approach to service delivery, which is focused on, and responsive to, women and their needs. This strategy is based on the goal of integrated maternity services delivered by a multi-disciplinary team with the "appropriate" professional determined based on need. In apparent deference to woman-centered care, the strategy avoids profession-centric terms, such as "midwifery led," which may unduly focus attention on the profession. This is problematic and may be viewed as unethical communication because the premise of woman-centered care emerged from the practice of midwifery, which is based on the principle of care offered in a woman-centered framework.[24] Midwifery shifts the power and control of decision-making back to the woman and may threaten an industrialized, medicalized model of healthcare driven by experts and reliant on standardization and efficiencies of practice.[25] Therefore, proposing woman-centered care while failing to elevate midwifery is at odds with the strategy's goals and with Irish tradition and culture.

HIQA's first monitoring program included inspections of maternity services in 2018 and 2019, and it found shortfalls and noncompliance with the national standards in a number of areas, including lack of maternity networks and formal care pathways, substandard infrastructure and physical environment, and inadequate midwifery staffing, among others.[26] Overall, HIQA noted that limited progress had been made to implement the National Maternity Strategy. The report identified numerous maternity units presenting an infection risk to women. Many services were provided by staff working unsafe rosters and overtime. A midwife we interviewed described the healthcare system as "bursting at the seams," and a physician we interviewed concurred: "We have a health care system that's literally on its knees." Although the National Maternity Strategy demanded that "all women must have access to standardized ultrasound services,"[27] a physician we interviewed said, "We still haven't gotten universal coverage with anatomy scans." Healthcare providers we interviewed also described lack of beds in hospitals, long gynecology waiting lists, lack of staff, and lack of clinic appointments.

A number of recent studies show that maternity services in Ireland continue to provide an obstetric consultant-led model of care, which is not woman-centered and lacks continuity of care.[28] According to a women's health activist, "We are a long way away from what we would consider a woman-centered model of reproductive care. There is real medicalization of childbirth with high Cesarean rates, almost no access to home births, and a very scornful attitude toward women who want home births." Indeed, a recent analysis of women's and clinicians' experiences found that woman-centered care is not routinely provided in Ireland.[29] Participants identified a lack of genuine choice and partnership in decision-making, highlighting healthcare providers' application of rules as inflexible, hierarchical, and disempowering.[30] Another study found that women's experiences of maternity services in Ireland were sporadic and failed to meet their needs.[31] These women described feeling unheard, unseen, and uncared for, needing streamlined information, relationship-based care, understanding of individual needs, and dedicated postnatal support.[32]

REPRODUCTIVE JUSTICE

The goal of *Healthy Ireland: A Framework for Improved Health and Wellbeing 2013–2025* is to improve the health and well-being of the people of Ireland.[33] Through a life-course approach, *Healthy Ireland* focuses on healthy behaviors throughout the entire life cycle, including pregnancy. The framework emphasizes that the social determinants of health, including economic, social, cultural, and environmental contexts, impact health outcomes. As a result, *Healthy Ireland* aims to provide holistic intervention and support starting with antenatal care that acknowledges the family's socioeconomic circumstances.

The socioeconomic position (SEP) of women giving birth in Ireland can be evaluated through the National Perinatal Reporting System, which uses occupation classification to define SEP. These data show that women in Ireland experience pregnancy-related healthcare disparities based on SEP. Mothers whose SEP was categorized as home duties or intermediate nonmanual workers made up the largest share of total births in 2013 (20.4% and 20%, respectively).[34] While the highest perinatal mortality rate was among the nonclassified group, mothers who reported home duties as their occupation represented the second highest perinatal mortality rate (9 per 1,000 births).[35] Mothers whose SEP was categorized as employers and managers, however, represented the lowest perinatal mortality rate (4.4 per 1,000 births).[36]

Women in Ireland also experience pregnancy-related healthcare disparities based on location. A recent study found that access to maternity services in Ireland varied significantly depending on geography, with rural areas offering minimal access to care.[37] Disparities have also been identified among pregnant women who are Travellers, immigrants, migrants, and asylum-seekers. Traveller women have a lower average age of childbirth compared to other women in Ireland.[38] According to Eithne Luibhéid, Travellers face racism that pathologizes their bodies, encouraging them to obtain genetic counseling prior to marriage and reproduction.[39] Women from European Union (EU) countries outside of Ireland accounted for 15.5% of births in Ireland in 2013, while women from non-EU countries represented 6.6% of births.[40] In 2014, mothers of newborns in Ireland were from over 110 countries.[41] Although Direct Provision offers migrants and asylum-seekers medical care, pregnant women in the system face unique barriers to antenatal, intrapartum, and postnatal care, including language barriers, lack of information, and challenges navigating the Irish healthcare system. According to Luibhéid, Direct Provision controls, contains, and incapacitates migrants, aiming to prevent illegal immigration and, ultimately, redefining nationalist sexual norms and racial, gender, economic, and geopolitical hierarchies.[42] Luibhéid describes how pregnancy, sexuality, and prevailing sexual norms impact migrants' likelihood of being defined as legal or illegal.[43] For example, until 2003, after giving birth to a child, migrant women were able to enter the Irish welfare system and live independently.[44]

Women facing infertility also experience unique challenges in Ireland. According to Jill Allison, infertility problematizes the moral, social, and political meanings of reproduction, which are inextricably linked to nature and biology.[45] This is evident in the limited medical treatment offered by Ireland's HSE to overcome infertility. Although medications and surgical treatments are available, assisted reproductive technology, including intrauterine insemination, in vitro fertilization (IVF), and intracytoplasmic sperm injection, are not covered by the public health service.[46] Medications used as part of fertility treatment may be covered by the Drugs Payment Scheme, and individuals may claim IVF costs through the tax relief for medical expenses scheme.[47] Evelyn Mahon and Noelle Cutter argue that a stigma is associated with infertility in Ireland, which may be reduced by raising awareness of infertility and offering eligible couples earlier access to IVF.[48]

The Children and Family Relationships Act of 2015 provides some protection for heterosexual and lesbian couples to take advantage of donor-assisted human reproduction (DAHR), including donor eggs and sperm. However, because there is no specific legislation addressing surrogacy in Ireland, it is unregulated, making it neither legal nor illegal. A 2021 review found that children's rights and best interests are served by recognizing intended family relationships in DAHR procedures, including surrogacy.[49] The review also recommended the expedient enactment of comprehensive legislation regulating surrogacy in Ireland.[50] Allison argues that nature serves as the foundation of the moral authority of the Church, political, and medical institutions in Ireland, which results in the overemphasis of genetics and biology in reproduction and conceptions of health and identity.[51] As a result, experiencing infertility treatment leads to dismissing religious tenets as obstructive and nature as inadequate, contesting accepted understandings of nature and biology and, ultimately, contravening the norms of reproduction.[52]

The campaign to repeal the Eighth Amendment illuminated healthcare disparities faced by women in Ireland beyond abortion. According to one scholar and activist we interviewed:

> The Eighth Amendment in itself was a form of reproductive violence just sitting there in the constitution because its effects were so widespread as far as for women who continued their pregnancies as well. Pregnancy just becomes something different in that context, I suppose that has an effect culturally but also on a personal level in terms of how you think about pregnancy and reproduction it is all just scary because it's not a safe place to be pregnant or give birth.

The women's health activists we talked with emphasized that while Ireland was "not a safe place to be pregnant or give birth" for all women, health disparities were exacerbated for vulnerable women. According to another scholar and activist we interviewed, "There are very gender-specific issues that intersect with issues of race and citizenship. And you have to be able to acknowledge that all women have forms of oppression, but there are women in certain positions who have very specific experiences of discrimination and oppression that need to be acknowledged." She went on to explain that "it's made me feel very differently about feminism because if it stops with the people who are exactly like you then it's just not feminism at all."

Still another scholar explained how the movement for repeal was grounded in reproductive justice and intersectionality:

> We're not just talking about the access to abortion, we're talking about the rights to have babies and the citizenship referendum, which directly targeted black mothers, women of African descent who were accused of baby tourism in Ireland. We also look at sterilizations, episiotomies, there's a whole history of attempts to control reproductive freedoms of people. It's only an intersectional feminist approach that will allow us to address it comprehensively.

Despite its limitations, the first National Maternity Strategy represents progress toward reproductive justice. Unfortunately, only months after HIQA's first monitoring program evaluating the implementation of the strategy, the COVID-19 pandemic emerged, further stressing the HSE. A National Public Health Emergency Team (NPHET) was activated in January 2020 to respond to the COVID-19 virus and work in unison with the HSE to implement regulations in response to the pandemic.[53] Scholars have identified a lack of women leaders and gender expertise on the NPHET, with a subcommittee for vulnerable groups excluding women's organizations, ethnic minorities, and migrants.[54] As a result, this approach negatively impacted the quality of women's health and healthcare experiences during the pandemic.

Government responses to COVID, including lockdowns, disproportionately impacted women's mental and physical health and financial stability.[55] Due to disruptions in access to reproductive and sexual health services, maternal mortality rates increased globally.[56] In addition, pregnant women face a higher risk of death from the COVID-19 virus, with a case fatality rate of 25%.[57] Women's mental and physical health suffered during the COVID-19 pandemic.[58]

Studies show women experienced increased depressive symptoms related to healthcare.[59] A multinational study including Ireland found high levels of depressive symptoms and generalized anxiety among pregnant and breastfeeding women.[60] Pregnant women in Ireland experienced lower perceived social support and increased stress during the pandemic.[61] A survey of Irish women found that 75% were negatively impacted by visitor restrictions in hospitals.[62] In Ireland, postpartum women reported not having their partner with them in the hospital as the main negative consequence of the restrictions.[63] Scholars therefore have called for an urgent re-evaluation of the Irish restrictions on partners in maternity care.[64]

As a result of COVID-19 hospital restrictions globally, women reported suffering discrimination and decreased overall satisfaction with healthcare.[65] Pregnant women with lower levels of education and limited access to information experienced higher rates of anxiety, which may impact health outcomes for mother and baby.[66] During the early months of the pandemic, EU states reported a 60% increase in emergency calls related to intimate partner violence.[67] Subsequent research confirmed an increase in domestic violence reports in Ireland, including calls to helplines and police reports.[68] A broad-based screening to identify depression in pregnant women during the COVID-19 pandemic found that medically sensitive women, women of color, and immigrants may be most in need of treatment to assist in coping and recovery from the pandemic.[69]

TRUTH-TELLING: IN OUR SHOES— COVID PREGNANCY

The *In Our Shoes—Covid Pregnancy* social media campaign is an example of contemporary reproductive justice activism and truth-telling in response to the COVID-19 restrictions in Ireland. *In Our*

Shoes shared women's experiences with maternal health services during the COVID-19 pandemic in Ireland. The campaign was created in September 2020 to shed light on the impact of healthcare restrictions in place since March 2020, which forced women to access Irish maternity services alone. As an introduction, the founders of the campaign wrote: "This is your body, your birth, your baby. Don't let restrictions erode what should be one of the most amazing experiences of your life. You are amazing, and you have got this. Don't be afraid, be informed, be empowered. We see you. We are you."[70] The campaign was active on Facebook (@inourshoescovidpregnancy) with 9,742 followers and on Instagram (@inourshoes_covidpregnancy) with 7,788 followers. *In Our Shoes* filled a gap in national discourse about emerging restrictions in maternity services. The campaign highlighted the lack of uniformity in hospital regulations and the lack of benchmarks for lifting restrictions, many of which remained in place as of September 2021.

Throughout the COVID-19 pandemic, healthcare institutions attempted to ensure the safety of pregnant people, infants, and staff from the virus through significant restrictions on maternity services, including prohibiting a companion during labor, limiting breastfeeding, and reducing contact between parents and infants. The *In Our Shoes* social media campaign collected anonymous narratives from women impacted by COVID-19 restrictions in Ireland and posted their stories online. Our analysis of these posts, described in the following section, revealed that the COVID-19 pandemic impacted women's experiences of pregnancy, labor, childbirth, and the postpartum period through the embodied experience, mental health, and lack of social support. The embodied experience of pregnancy and delivery during the pandemic resulted in increased iatrogenic harms and disruptions in care. Women's mental health was impacted by restrictions on maternal-infant attachment; feelings of anxiety, fear, guilt, and loneliness; and trauma. The pandemic disrupted women's social support by failing to respect women's chosen labor companion and forcing women to face loss alone. This analysis suggests that maternity restrictions may be defined as obstetric violence and understood as part of a long history of the Irish Church-state's attempt to control and repress women. It also revealed the need for systemic change to ensure every woman's right to high-quality, respectful maternity care.

IN OUR SHOES—COVID PREGNANCY

The *In Our Shoes—Covid Pregnancy* case study also provides an example of the ways that the Irish state-Church coalition and medical profession continue to regulate women's reproductive lives and engage in systematic repression during labor and childbirth.[71] Throughout the COVID-19 pandemic, as already mentioned, pregnant people faced increased restrictions on maternity services, including the exclusion of companions during labor and birth.[72] Since March 2020, over 120,000 people accessing maternity care and their families have been impacted by restrictions in Ireland. Although these restrictions were, as also already mentioned, attempts to ensure the safety of pregnant people, infants, and staff from COVID-19,[73] these regulations are antithetical to human rights in childbirth and the right to have a chosen companion during labor and childbirth, including during the COVID-19 pandemic. According to the World Health Organization (WHO), the COVID-19 pandemic magnified existing health systems issues and disrupted access to maternal health services, resulting in women not receiving needed care, which may create life-long consequences.[74]

On World Patient Safety Day, September 17, 2021, the WHO focused on safe maternal and newborn care and called on stakeholders to "act now for safe and respectful childbirth." Highlighting how the COVID-19 pandemic exacerbated disparities in quality health services, the WHO argued that "since maternity care is also affected by issues of gender equity and violence, women's experiences during childbirth have the potential to either empower them or inflict damage and emotional trauma."[75] In response, the International Federation of Gynaecology and Obstetrics (FIGO) released an Ethical Framework for Respectful Maternity Care During Pregnancy and Childbirth that emphasized the importance of maternity care as a partnership between healthcare providers and the "MotherBaby-Family" that is value-based, individualized, and supportive.[76]

There is growing evidence that changes to healthcare delivery designed to protect patients and staff from COVID-19 may lead to harmful consequences for maternal health.[77] Scholars argue that COVID-19 restrictions during childbirth are unnecessary, not evidence-based, disrespectful of human dignity, and deny women's human rights.[78] Research shows that COVID-19 maternity restrictions are inconsistently applied, not grounded in evidence or human rights, and may increase long-term adverse psychological, physical, and emotional outcomes among women, newborns, and families.[79] Michelle Sadler, Gonzalo Leiva, and Ibone Olza suggest that the COVID-19 restrictions during childbirth, including prohibition of a companion during labor, unnecessary interventions, immediate separation of mother and newborn, and the prevention of breastfeeding, are obstetric violence.[80]

Throughout the COVID-19 pandemic, the WHO advocated for every woman's right to high-quality, respectful maternity care during labor, delivery, and the postpartum period.[81] Meeting this standard requires respecting the emotional, practical, and health benefits of a chosen labor companion and accommodating women's supportive companion. A consensus statement of midwifery organizations defined factors that disrupt normal physiologic childbirth and cause iatrogenic harm related to interventions during labor. These factors include induction or augmentation of labor; an unsupportive environment (i.e., bright lights, cold room, lack of privacy, multiple providers, lack of supportive companions, etc.); time constraints, including those driven by institutional policy and/or staffing; nutritional deprivation (e.g., food and drink); opiates, regional analgesia, or general anesthesia; episiotomy; operative vaginal or abdominal birth; immediate cord clamping; separation of mother and infant; and/or any situation in which the mother feels threatened or unsupported.[82] In August 2021, the Midwives Association of Ireland called on the HSE and government to acknowledge the impact of ongoing restrictions on those accessing maternity care and argued "it is now critical that we urgently focus on every woman's human right to have respectful and dignified care."[83]

We performed a qualitative content analysis to analyze 134 publicly available online posts from the *In Our Shoes* social media campaign shared between September 2020 and September 2021. Irish women were invited to submit their stories to the campaign's administrators, and all narratives were posted anonymously. We collected all anonymous testimonials posted during the study period to determine the impact of restrictions on pregnant people's birthing experiences. As of September 2021, 90% of all adults were vaccinated in Ireland, and most day-to-day restrictions had been lifted. The #BetterMaternityCare campaign called on the Minister for Health to end all partner restrictions across Irish Maternity Services. This analysis also offers insight to improve women's autonomy and decision-making power in healthcare after the pandemic.[84]

The COVID-19 pandemic impacted women's embodied experiences of pregnancy, labor, childbirth, and the postpartum period. The embodied experience of pregnancy and delivery during the pandemic resulted in increased iatrogenic harms, which encompass factors that disrupt normal physiological birth and include interventions or augmentations of labor. Most narratives described an unsupportive environment, including a lack of privacy, multiple providers, and lack of supportive companions. Many narratives described feeling coerced to accept interventions, including induction or augmentation of labor, analgesia, or cesarean birth in order to maintain access to their birth partner. For example, one woman wrote: "I was retraumatised all over again. I was repeatedly asked why I 'just didn't say no' to the midwife breaking my waters (despite her threatening to take my partner away; I was coerced and felt I had no choice but to say 'yes')."[85] Many stories revealed how companion restrictions limited patient advocacy through coercion. Uniformly, these narratives uncovered iatrogenic harm through situations in which the mother felt threatened or unsupported.

Women also described disruptions in care, including cancellations of appointments and follow-up appointments, difficulty making appointments, poor patient care, multiple women in the same room, and inability to bring clothes and items to the hospital. One woman described her experience sharing a room with four other new mothers, including one who had a COVID-19 exposure before entering the hospital. She wrote: "In the hours after giving birth, I was left in the room alone with my baby who was barely 1 day old, the room was overcrowded with broken machines (for checking your vitals) and the toilets had jugs of peoples urine and blood sitting there all day."[86] Women's stories described the embodied experience of perinatal care during COVID-19, including vomiting in pain and bleeding without being able to access a shower, clean clothes, water, food, or the opportunity to clean their babies.

During the pandemic, women's mental health during pregnancy, labor, childbirth, and the postpartum period was impacted by restrictions on maternal-infant attachment. Many women experienced iatrogenic harm through the separation of mother and infant immediately after birth, with limited visitation in the postpartum period, negatively impacting the maternal-infant bonding process. One woman commented on the pain of this isolation: "I never got skin-to-skin, despite making my intention to breastfeed known. The first face my baby saw, the first hands that held her, were those of the midwife who has ruined my life."[87] Women who had newborns in the neonatal intensive care unit (NICU) experienced increased restrictions and time constraints driven by institutional policy. Many women described visiting hours restricted to as little as two hours per day. In some cases, time constraints in the NICU meant separating parents from their dying infants. One mother posted: "4 babies didn't make it home during our time in NICU and every mother said the same thing 'they took away most of the time I could have had with my baby by limiting parents time in the unit.' "[88]

For many women, accessing maternity services during COVID-19 led to feelings of anxiety, fear, guilt, and loneliness. Women discussed mistreatment during prenatal care, labor, delivery, and the postpartum period. Some women continue to experience feelings of helplessness and guilt because they were separated from their infants. According to one woman, "I have so much guilt for the time I lost with him, not knowing he wouldn't make it. The loneliness, isolation and anxiety the restrictions have caused. I still struggle to go outside by myself most of the time. The mental & emotional toll of not having my partner with me and the guilt of not being with my baby 24/7 will be with me forever."[89]

Many women described the perinatal care they received under COVID-19 restrictions as traumatic. One woman shared that for her and her husband, the experience "broke us."[90] Women described facing emotional abandonment and neglect in hospitals. Many women described feeling isolated and talked down to by staff. One woman shared her trauma, writing: "I was so scared the whole time and genuinely thought I was going to die on my own. 4 months on, and my head is a mess. I'm so traumatized by the whole experience. I had nobody to hold my hand or wipe my tears. I was terrified. No woman should be alone for this."[91] Many women described long-term mental health consequences of birthing during COVID-19. For some, this experience negatively impacted their desire to have more children. One woman wrote: "I will never have another child. Even if I could conceive naturally, I wouldn't after my experience in the hospital."[92] Unfortunately, this experience is not unique to the COVID-19 restrictions. A study of women's experiences of childbirth in Ireland prior to the pandemic found that some women reported they would not have another baby as a result of their childbirth experiences.[93]

The pandemic disrupted women's social support during pregnancy, labor, childbirth, and the postpartum period by failing to respect women's chosen labor companion. Most of the women in this study were separated from their companion of choice during prenatal care, labor, delivery, and the postpartum period. Many women described enduring cesarean sections alone and their partners being unable to meet the new baby for days. Other women endured pain and coercive interventions to ensure their partners could be present for childbirth. When an epidural wasn't working for one woman, she chose light sedation, feeling the pain of cesarean section in order to keep her companion during delivery. Giving birth without a companion of choice led to feelings of isolation for many woman. One woman wrote: "Covid robbed me of my birth joy. Birth is unpredictable and difficult, and I think I would have been able to endure that had I had my partner to help me through it. I'm recovering now at home, but processing the sadness took weeks."[94] This shows that lacking a companion of choice can have a lasting impact even after birth.

In Ireland, approximately 14,000 couples, or about one in five pregnancies, experience spontaneous miscarriage.[95] The National Maternity Strategy identifies best practices for women who experience miscarriage or receive bad news during pregnancy, including being cared for in a private room away from other pregnant women or newborns. A recent analysis of ten publicly available Irish national health service–commissioned inquiry reports relating to perinatal deaths and pregnancy loss services published between 2005 and 2018 found that bereavement care was not consistently respectful.[96] In some situations, patient autonomy was disregarded, including instances when staff were dishonest or failed to offer all management options during labor or early pregnancy loss.[97] The authors of this analysis suggested that failing to accommodate different factors, such as patients' language or culture, negatively impacted communication with bereaved parents.[98]

Many women faced bad news alone during prenatal care, labor, delivery, and the postpartum period. COVID-19 restrictions required women to enter diagnostic appointments and termination procedures alone, forcing women to carry the emotional burden of this news on their own throughout the pandemic. One woman described her experience: "My beautiful baby is gone. I'm all alone. I'm all alone. No one to tell me it's not my fault, or no one to tell me it will be ok. No one to hold me tight." Many women who required treatment after miscarriage described how COVID-19 altered standard care in disturbing ways, including changes in anesthesia.

Women described COVID-19 restrictions in maternity care as sexist, barbaric, and unfair. Many women suggested that regulations were part of a long history of the government's attempt to control women. According to one woman, "How can women's mental and physical health YET AGAIN be forgotten about, not even last on the agenda, not on the agenda at all."[99] Many women described inconsistent regulations that disproportionately impacted birthing women. Other participants shared discrepancies in the same hospital's policy regarding companions. Another woman who had a history of miscarriage shared how, while waiting alone for her thirteen-week scan, she was approached in the hospital by a television producer recruiting participants to appear on a new show filming there. She wrote: "It's really offensive and it's morally wrong."[100] Women shared that maternity restrictions during the COVID-19 pandemic revealed inherent failings in maternal and child care and called for systemic change. One woman wrote: "The whole maternity service in Ireland needs an overhaul if we are ever to really see women being treated with respect and have real autonomy over our bodies and how we give birth."[101]

CONCLUSION

The COVID-19 pandemic impacted women's experiences of pregnancy, labor, childbirth, and the postpartum period through the embodied experience, mental health, and lack of social support. The embodied experience of pregnancy and delivery during the pandemic resulted in increased iatrogenic harms and disruptions in care. During the pandemic, women's mental health was impacted by restrictions on maternal-infant attachment and by feelings of anxiety, fear, guilt, and loneliness, and trauma. The pandemic disrupted women's social support by failing to respect women's chosen labor companion, forcing women to face loss alone, and revealing the need for systemic change to ensure every woman's right to high-quality, respectful maternity care.

It is clear, however, that the pandemic exacerbated failings of the maternity system that were already evident. Shortly before the pandemic, Nadine Edwards, Rosemary Mander, and Jo Murphy-Lawless described Ireland's maternity services as being in a state of emergency.[102] They accurately predicted that institutional, regulatory, political, and governmental decisions would continue to negatively impact the ability of midwives to care for their patients and result in adverse health outcomes for pregnant women.[103] Most of the women in our analysis were separated from their companion of choice during prenatal care, labor, delivery, and the postpartum period. Other women endured pain and coercive interventions to ensure their partners could be present for childbirth.

Women faced disruptions in care and increased iatrogenic harms, including lack of supportive companions and feeling coerced to accept interventions, such as induction or augmentation of labor, analgesia, or cesarean birth. Women described an unsupportive environment, including a lack of privacy, multiple providers, separation of mother an infant, and other situations in which the mother felt threatened or unsupported. For many women, accessing maternity services led to feelings of anxiety, fear, guilt, and loneliness. Many women described the perinatal care they received as traumatic and struggled with long-term mental health consequences of birthing during COVID-19. Prior research described how the Irish Church-state coalition merged with an institutionalized, medicalized model of healthcare to enact obstetric violence in the twentieth century.[104] This chapter contributes to research finding that the COVID-19 pandemic maternity restrictions may be understood as obstetric violence encompassing the medicalization of childbirth and unnecessary or forced medical interventions.[105]

Many women suggested that COVID-19 regulations were part of a long history of the government's attempt to control women. In 2020, a HIQA analysis of the national standards for better maternity services revealed shortfalls and noncompliance with the national standards in a number of areas, including lack of maternity networks and formal care pathways, among others.[106] On August 11, 2021, the Midwives Association of Ireland argued against ongoing restrictions in maternity care and urged the government to consider the input of stakeholders, including public representative groups. Scholars have examined the indirect effects of the COVID-19 pandemic and identified women as particularly vulnerable to the impact of amplifying existing health inequalities, arguing that these issues should be a priority for recovery programs during and after the pandemic.[107]

In Ireland, although the exclusion of women's expertise from the pandemic response created negative gendered impacts, feminist responses to the pandemic were innovative, inclusive, and independent.[108] Pauline Cullen and Mary Murphy argue that Ireland responded to the COVID-19 crisis in nimble and innovative ways, which offers an opportunity for feminists to move beyond the traditionally slow pace of gendered social change to achieve social transformation.[109]

This analysis shows that pregnant people faced increased iatrogenic harms during the COVID-19 pandemic. This chapter suggests that maternity restrictions may be defined as obstetric violence and understood as part of a long history of the Irish Church-state's attempt to control and repress women. The *In Our Shoes—Covid Pregnancy* social media campaign revealed the continued need for systemic change to ensure every woman's right to high-quality, respectful maternity care. In addition, the campaign highlighted the importance of women sharing their story to highlight the gendered effects of COVID-19 and to achieve social transformation as Ireland recovers from the pandemic.

Childbirth

Mary Harris Jones was born in 1837 in Cork, Ireland, and moved to North America when she was 10 years old. She was later known as Mother Jones and called "the most dangerous woman in America" because of her advocacy on behalf of workers' rights. Upton Sinclair fictionalized Mother Jones in *The Coal War*,[1] describing her weapons as "stories" that ignited the "flame of protest" and revolt. In the United States, *Mother Jones* is the oldest investigative news organization in the nation, training emerging investigative story-tellers and aiming for reporting that inspires change. In Ireland, the Cork Mother Jones Committee honors individuals who fight for human rights and social justice. The 2021 Spirit of Mother Jones Award recognized the Cork Survivors and Supporters Alliance (CSSA), which campaigned for the memorialization of the women and children buried on the grounds of the former Mother and Baby Home at Bessborough in Cork. According to Abby Bender, 75% of the babies born at Bessborough in 1943 died within a year.[2] The 2021 award acknowledged the CSSA's "bravery and determination," as well as "their efforts to organize a voice for the mothers of deceased children."[3] The continued need for grassroots organizing and truth-telling to preserve human rights highlights the connections between women's health scandals throughout Irish history.

Catching Fire. Beth Sundstrom and Cara Delay, Oxford University Press. © Oxford University Press 2023.
DOI: 10.1093/oso/9780197743942.003.0006

The legacy of the culture that produced Ireland's Mother and Baby Homes continues to impact the gender health gap and women's experiences of reproductive health and childbirth. First, pro-natalist attitudes persist amidst continued problems accessing contraception and abortion; Ireland maintains one of the highest fertility rates in Europe at 1.82 children per woman in 2016.[4] Furthermore, the medicalization of childbirth and the power of physicians, which has denied women birthing choices and autonomy, persevere. Since 2007, for example, the proportion of women undergoing cesarean section in Ireland continues to increase. In 2020, 35.4% of women delivered by cesarean section.[5] Although the rates of cesarean section have increased since 2000 in many developed countries, the Organisation for Economic Co-operation and Development (OECD) average rate is 28% of live births.[6] According to the World Health Organization (WHO), when cesarean section rates rise above 10%, there is no improvement in maternal or newborn mortality rates. The WHO's global guidelines to inform evidence-based, nonclinical interventions to reduce cesarean section rates stated: "The sustained, unprecedented rise in caesarean section rates is a major public health concern. There is an urgent need for evidence-based guidance to address the trend."[7]

This chapter explores the historical, social, and cultural origins and impacts of the medicalization and institutionalization of childbirth in Ireland. Although 99% of women in Ireland give birth in a hospital,[8] the COVID-19 pandemic and restrictions in maternity care led to a 30% increase in homebirths nationally.[9] Scholars argue that hospital births undermine the social rite of birth by privileging medical authority and undermining women's bodily experience.[10] The constructed normalcy of hospital birth is supported by media, physicians, prenatal classes, and a culture that fuels women's fears and desires for a safe birth. However, there is a global attempt to reject the pathologizing of birth and promote humanistic, midwifery-led care, one that is supported by the WHO and by Irish activists and advocates. This chapter explores the history of the biomedical model of childbirth in Ireland in the twentieth century; the history and current status of reproductive justice activism, particularly birthing options, focusing on interviews with current activists and medical professionals; and the campaign for the Coroners (Amendment) Act 2019 led by the Elephant Collective, which provides evidence of an activist group that achieved success in effecting change at the state level.

REPRODUCTIVE JUSTICE

Contemporary organizing and coalition-building to raise the voices of women impacted by health scandals in Ireland build on a long history of truth-telling. Current reproductive justice activism evolved from the foundation of women's rights advocacy in the 1970s and earlier. Indeed, many of today's campaigners had been involved in the women's rights movement for decades. According to a legal expert and activist we interviewed:

> I think that the intergenerational dimension of Repeal can't be underestimated . . . . Repeal was about what it is to be a woman in Ireland—and as part of the global research of feminist discourse—are women going to put up with being spoken about and treated in this way? . . . I think Repeal was one of those places where people were kind of taking stock of their own childbirth experiences if they had them, their relationships with their mothers and grandmothers and so on, and really kind of taking stock of that question.

Another scholar and activist described how the success of Repeal raised the profile of women's voices:

There are so many women who have spoken out in public, who have incredible leadership and are very inspiring and I think that's changed the way people think about involvement in public life ... People can positively influence the democratic process— they can make it work—for what they view as positive change.

An analysis of the archives of Attic Press reveal a feminist commitment to intersectionality beginning in the 1970s that would be intrinsic to the modern reproductive justice movement. Róisín Conroy was an activist and campaigner for women's rights in Ireland, as well as the co-founder of Attic Press, a feminist publishing house. She collected the Attic Press archives, which are housed in the Boole Library, University College Cork. An entry in the *Rebel Women* magazine demonstrates a commitment to the core principle of intersectionality: "While one of us is oppressed—we are all oppressed."[11] Echoing the current struggles in maternity services, documents from 1978 describe the need for more research on childbirth conducted with birthing mothers to better understand their treatment in medical care. In a 1970s meeting of Irish Women United (12, Pembroke Street, Dublin 2), women discussed the same issues that campaigners contend with today: "Irish governments have consistently ignored the rights of women ... The days the government and church took all the important decisions concerning our lives, our bodies, our sexuality, our employment situation, with the slightest consideration of our needs are numbered."[12] This meeting also foreshadowed reproductive justice as a human right, which necessitates a social safety net with government providing the basic necessities that parents need to raise their children in safe and healthy environments, including housing and childcare. According to Irish Women United, "when we decide to have children we want proper housing, childcare facilities, creches, nurseries in the places we work and live in."[13] More recently, scholars have argued that women-centered maternity care must incorporate quality healthcare during pregnancy and birth, as well as postpartum support services in the community, such as affordable infant care.[14] In 1977, the Women's International Information and Communication Service Conference identified the ultimate goal of reproductive justice and the necessity to "study the changes involved in passing from a patriarchal and authoritarian system to a system of equals, in which women will not be assimilated into a man's world, but which, instead, will be a new society in which values which up until now have been repressed will be respected."[15]

In the current women's health movement, interviews with activists revealed a common understanding of intersectionality and reproductive justice at the core of the movement. In an interview with a member of the Irish Family Planning Association (IFPA), the interviewee remembered a training in Ireland by SisterSong, the largest national multiethnic reproductive justice collective in the United States:

> When SisterSong came and was talking about the issues around decisions around motherhood, and we could point to some historic scandals that have happened in Irish maternity hospitals ... Organizations like AIMS [Association for Improvements in the Maternity Services] Ireland recounted women's experiences of decision making within maternity hospitals. Of course, the focus on this is happening to women, reproductive healthcare in particular, and women with disabilities, I think those voice[s] became important during the campaign . . . Just a couple of weeks before the vote, there was controversy around CervicalCheck, there's maternal death cases, as well ... so I think we took what SisterSong was saying, we took that idea of reproductive justice, being more than abortion rights, being one part of reproductive justice, and broadened it, and I think that resonated with people.

Zakiya Luna describes the global connections SisterSong made with women and organizations beyond the United States, suggesting that "another way SisterSong's idea of global responsibility emerged was in its claim to represent women globally and its sometimes stated goal of doing so."[16]

A legal scholar and activist we interviewed described how Lawyers for Choice incorporated reproductive justice into their campaign for Repeal:

> The law currently is about reproductive control and reproductive justice would mean an overcoming and a shedding of those kinds of mechanisms of intervention, surveillance, distrust, pressure, coercion and so on. So for us, in Lawyers for Choice, we used reproductive justice as a way of saying there's an aspiration for law, which of course will always be kind of imperfectly achieved but there is nevertheless an aspiration that law would be able to do more than prohibit and restrain, so I think that's probably the sense in which we were inspired by that kind of idea.

Many activists agreed that a focus on reproductive justice and intersectionality pushed the movement to expand beyond abortion rights. One interviewed scholar reflected:

> An overt embrace of intersectionality that brought attention to reproductive justice in Ireland . . . became a frame for us to explain what we do . . . I think that's what intersectional feminism is to a lot of us, that we aren't staying in a narrow bend of abortion rights, but reproductive justice is something much more broadly conceived of.

As another scholar activist said:

So from my perspective, it was really intersectional and it really spread out and touched so many people from so many different backgrounds. It was really refreshing to see people come together and have a common ground for work, so in that way it was very intersectional.

For many activists, the current reproductive justice movement reflected the human rights concerns of campaigners in the 1970s. One activist described the legacy of Repeal:

It does suggest that there are other campaigns that can be won, and inevitably some people have other ideas. For some people it's ending Church control of education, for others it's homelessness which is obviously huge, and I do see a lot more publicity around Direct Provision than I have ever seen before . . . I think that there is a momentum . . . I think people are quite inspired by the idea that they can effect change and put things onto the political agenda.

Most activists acknowledged the struggles around women's reproductive health as a class issue, as well as pointing to the ways that the current healthcare system marginalizes refugees and asylum-seekers, migrants, Travellers, and women of color. Still, many activists believed that the national movement could have embraced a more intersectional reproductive justice approach by consciously lifting up diverse voices, including women of color.

TRUTH-TELLING

In early 2019, an activist we interviewed described the tragic death of Karen McEvoy who died of sepsis on Christmas Day 2018 after giving birth at the Coombe Women & Infants University Hospital. She said:

> In recent weeks there's been a horrific story about a maternal death that happened on Christmas Day and there's more conversation again about the care that was provided but also more talk about how there's no mandatory inquest about maternal death in Ireland and we're failing to learn from what's happening, so I think there's a lot more critique and concern around maternity care . . . You see in these particular situations its often up to the family to fight and argue for these things but the families shouldn't be the ones that have to push for this. Like all evidence based medicine you need to learn from when things go wrong.

Since 2013, the Elephant Collective, an homage to the herd that protects female elephants while giving birth, has led a national conversation about women who died in maternity services and the lack of mandatory inquests in Ireland. An activist and advocacy group including educators, birth activists, midwives, students, and families affected by maternal deaths, the Elephant Collective began raising awareness about the eight women who died in Irish maternity services between 2008 and 2014 whose deaths were investigated, as well as those whose deaths were unknown. The inquests into the deaths of those eight women resulted in verdicts of medical misadventure, which indicates an unintended outcome, such as a complication arising from a medical procedure or medication, but does not imply blame. According to the Maternal Death Enquiry Team, between 2011 and 2013, out of at least 27 maternal deaths, only three inquests were held.[17]

The Elephant Collective began commemorating the deaths of women in Irish maternity services through a multimedia exhibition, including a documentary *Picking up the Threads* by Anne-Marie Greene and a knitted quilt with over 100 contributors. Through feminist praxis, including knitting, painting, film, and other art, the Elephant Collective successfully raised awareness of the need for mandatory inquests. According to Dr. Jo Murphy-Lawless, who created the Collective with her midwifery students at Trinity College Dublin, "Irish women have had to live with the consequences of unchallenged medical authority bolstered by a state that refused to intervene until women pushed for action."[18] With no funding and no paid staff, women's health activists once again employed truth-telling to inspire legal change to improve healthcare services. Then-Teachta Dála (Member of Irish Parliament) Clare Daly, now Member of European Parliament, championed the Coroners (Amendment) Act 2019 and acknowledged the "heroic struggle" of the bereaved, "whose human tragedies have been turned into a movement to change the law . . . by the families of the women who died in maternity hospitals."[19] According to Martina Hynan, this national campaign made maternal deaths visible in a scientific model of birth that renders the mother's body and experience of childbirth hidden and where the maternal body and maternal death is contested medically, socially, culturally, and politically.[20]

On January 12, 2018, Migrants and Ethnic-minorities for Reproductive Justice (MERJ) posted on Facebook:

> Another migrant woman of colour killed in a maternity hospital in Ireland: "The court was told what had happened was a 'cascade of negligence' in which one individual act of negligence was followed by another." Malak Thawley's case is absolutely horrific and our deepest sympathies go out to her family. This is why it is not enough to just #Repealthe8th. We must fight for #ReproductiveJustice![21]

Malak Thawley died at Dublin's National Maternity Hospital during surgery for an ectopic pregnancy. A coroner found she died by medical misadventure. In an interview with the *Irish Times*, Solicitor Caoimhe Haughey, who represented Malak's widower, said the "default position of the HSE [Health Service Executive] in a maternal death is to delay, deny and defend."[22]

In July 2019, approximately six months after Karen McEvoy's death, the Coroners (Amendment) Act was signed into law by the Presidential Commission.[23] The Act ensures public inquests are mandatory for all maternal deaths or late maternal deaths. According to Murphy-Lawless, "the Irish state has harmed women time and again. The new Coroners Act finally holds the state to account on the most violent of harms, causing a woman's death in childbirth."[24] P. Scranton and G. McNaull argue that the government should establish a Charter for the Bereaved, in consultation with families, advocacy groups, and campaign organizations, in order to prevent recurrence by ensuring narrative verdict recommendations identify systemic, institutional practices, and recurring deficiencies that contribute to a death.[25]

The first maternal death following the implementation of the Act was Nayyab Tariq, who died in Mayo University Hospital in March 2020. Nayyab died of postpartum hemorrhage and shock, and her inquest concluded with a verdict of medical misadventure. On October 7, 2021, responding to the verdict, Murphy-Lawless posted on behalf of the Elephant Collective:

> When are these crumbling, archaic, outmoded, arrogant, unaccountable maternity services going to come clean, own up, drop their contempt towards us and show Irish women the level of care and respect we require? There are individual midwives and clinicians within these services who desperately want to see change. Long promised, always deferred. These failing services

cannot be left room to hide any longer. This is why mandatory inquests are critically important.[26]

Through the Digital Repository of Ireland, the Elephant Collective will archive the campaign that successfully demanded mandatory inquests for all maternal deaths.

ADDRESSING THE MATERNITY CRISIS: MAKING CHILDBIRTH A POSITIVE EXPERIENCE

Scholars have identified a crisis in the Irish Maternity System.[27] Recent failures in maternity care provide evidence of the continuing influence of paternalistic, hierarchical healthcare that fails to center women's well-being.[28] A physician we interviewed said, "We have a health care system that's literally on its knees." The maternity mortality and morbidity crisis in Ireland must be understood in the historical context of institutionalization in Mother and Baby Homes, creating a legacy of social and cultural medicalization and pathologizing of women's bodies. The social and cultural impact of this history continues to impact the gender health gap, including underfunded maternity services that impact women's experiences of childbirth. An analysis of childbirth at the Coombe Hospital between the 1960s and 2010s found an increased rate of labor induction, instrumental delivery, and third-degree tears.[29] The rate of epidurals increased from 3.4% in the 1980s to 40.3% in 2010s.[30]

According to Jane X in a 2019 MERJ blog post, "Ireland has a legacy of institutional impunity and a history of women being repressed and controlled which still reflects on its health care system practices."[31] An activist told us her childbirth story from twenty-eight years ago, and it reflected many of the same experiences that women in the *In Our Shoes—Covid Pregnancy* campaign shared about their contemporary experiences of childbirth in Ireland. She said:

> I encountered maternity services here through the eyes of somebody with no money, really young, in [Dublin], experiencing . . . what it's like to be a woman in this city, 28 years ago . . . I went to the Coombe "lying-in" hospital as it was once called . . . it was the height of the HIV problem, as they saw it, and the ward was full of beds of women who were really vulnerable, we were all vulnerable because of our age, lack of ability to pay anything, all in the public system, none of us were in a private room, none of us had flowers in our cups. I remember a nurse pulling a curtain, the woman opposite of me was probably 18, and saying "pulling the curtain" and that was the privacy you had, the curtain was pulled and saying to the woman, well you know you're HIV positive . . .
>
> It was just, there were loads of issues, let me say, with my baby. I was trying to feed my baby, loads of issues with that, and no one else was feeding the baby so my baby was crying and it was difficult. There was no holistic care, and the woman next to me, forget my breastfeeding activities. Everyone on the ward now knows she has HIV, and she has to know now whether her beautiful baby has it, it's not my business. It was a horrible position. So there we are, stuffed in this room, and we were treated quite badly. I remember going to the toilet, I had an epidural for the baby, and being given a bed pan, because you were paralyzed. Step in the bed pan and just left there, they didn't even tell me to press the thing. So I was on the bed pan for three hours before my baby starts screaming, and I had been trying to get someone to pay attention. It's like, I'm in a good place, here's me, chosen to have my baby, really happy with the place that I'm in, of course I have no money, but I can get some eventually . . . It was just a

horrible place to be, there was no care or attention paid to any of us. That was my first encounter and that was the cliff's edge as far as I'm concerned.

Later, when this activist became pregnant again, she reflected on the hypocrisy of a pro-natalist country that links women's value with childbearing and motherhood while failing to provide support. She said, "I can't believe I'm having baby number two in a country that tells me it cherishes all children equally, loves women, loves having babies, and does nothing for me. Just abandons you, doesn't help you feed the baby, have the baby, doesn't look after you in any way." Women's experiences in maternity care demonstrate how the well-known "architecture of containment" apparent in Magdalene laundries and Mother and Baby Homes shaped the evolution of the maternity care system in the twentieth century.[32] Hospitals, too, were part of the "architecture of containment," where women's bodies were surveilled and controlled, and where women's voices were obscured.

Nadine Edwards describes Irish maternity services as an institutionalized, medicalized, and fragmented system of maternity care that silences women's voices.[33] According to Mavis Kirkham, centralizing maternity services in hospitals created a commercial model of care, producing economies of scale by standardizing a series of tasks rather than supporting relationships to nurture women's self-confidence.[34] Rosemary Mander describes an obstetric culture of fear.[35] In an online survey by the Birth Project Group, midwives recounted unmanageable workloads and high levels of stress due to low staffing, leading to mental and physical illness that, ultimately, created unsafe care for birthing women.[36] In "Untangling the Maternity Crisis," Edwards, Mander, and Murphy-Lawless discuss the hostile environment in contemporary Irish maternity services, arguing that midwifery offers a woman-centered and community-based approach to improve childbirth.[37] A midwife shared with us the impact of capitalism on the quality of maternity care in Ireland:

> I suppose what I would feel really strongly about is, in terms of maternity services in Ireland is when we compare ourselves to the UK which is NHS [National Health Service] based, therefore when you're looking at total accuracy across the board where there isn't money to be made, then you see that midwives are at the floor of providing care and midwifery led services are pushed as the best options because they're cheaper and women have better outcomes, and when there's . . . obstetric dominance because the obstetricians are the ones that are making money off of it and we're basically limiting women's choice, we're not providing internationally best standard care practice, which is midwifery led care. That's the most frustrating thing for me I think.

Research shows that many women in Ireland feel anxious and alone during childbirth, but midwives play a critical role in empowering women to achieve a positive birth experience.[38] As we discuss in chapter 6, however, the roles and voices of midwives have been diminished historically. Scholars and practitioners have countered the dominant narrative of medicalization of childbirth by identifying the social, economic, and political systems that privilege medical authority and safety over women's lived experiences.

The Universal Declaration of Human Rights affirms that all women have the right to make autonomous decisions about their own bodies, including during labor and childbirth.[39] Women's childbirth experiences have long-term consequences for their health and well-being, as well as the health of their children and families.[40] Studies show that maternal dissatisfaction with childbirth may be related to routine obstetrical interventions, including labor augmentation and unplanned cesarean delivery.[41] At the Coombe

Hospital, the cesarean section rate rose from 5.9% in the 1960s to 29.7% in the 2010s.[42] Although there was not a significant change in the number of uterine ruptures, the rate of vaginal births after cesarean section dropped from 90.4% to 28.2%.[43] In partnership with Lamaze International, Coalition for Improving Maternity Services, and Childbirth Connection, among others, the WHO is working to reduce the number of cesarean deliveries in the United States and Western Europe. The National Institute for Health and Care Excellence (NICE), which provides recommendations to improve healthcare in the United Kingdom and is endorsed by the National Health Service, offers guidance on cesarean deliveries. The quality standard outlines the risks of cesarean delivery and aims to increase access to information and improve women's decision-making process.[44] In a recent study of Irish maternity units, researchers found that women with private healthcare coverage were more likely to experience an obstetric intervention, including cesarean delivery, surgical vaginal delivery, episiotomy, induction of labor, and epidural anesthesia, even after controlling for risk factors.[45] The Maternal Health and Maternal Morbidity in Ireland (MAMMI) study found that first-time mothers in private care were twice as likely to have a cesarean section compared with those choosing public maternity services.[46] Private care also led to an increased likelihood of epidural anesthesia and longer postpartum hospital stays.[47]

Women's satisfaction with childbirth is integrally linked to shared decision-making and the ability to exercise informed choice.[48] Scholars argue that the quality of maternity care must be measured beyond safety and mortality and morbidity outcomes to include women's experiences and psychological and emotional well-being.[49] The MAMMI study found that risk status did not influence choice of maternity care pathway (e.g., public vs. private); however, those at higher risk experienced poorer outcomes across all five indicators of birth experience (autonomy, pain relief, maternal confidence, second baby intention, and breastfeeding).[50] In a recent study of Irish clinicians, researchers found that increasing rates of vaginal birth after cesarean delivery could be achieved by fostering shared decision-making, which relies on rapport, trust, and unbiased information.[51] Understanding women's values, beliefs, and attitudes is central to offering woman-centered care in order to improve women's childbirth experiences and birth outcomes.[52] In addition, research points to the conclusion that women desire more information and increased control of the childbirth experience.[53] Improving women's satisfaction in childbirth requires empowering women with information, including the risks and benefits of interventions, to take control of labor and delivery by making informed choices through shared decision-making.[54]

In a recent study, women's preferences for childbirth experiences included the availability of pain relief, individualized care, and partnership with a midwife.[55] Women described their ideal birth experience as being as natural as possible; however, they rejected the dichotomy between natural and medicalized care and preferred "the best of both worlds."[56] A physician we interviewed described the need to move beyond polarized "natural" versus "technological" childbirth:

> Birth became very medialized and very regimented and there was a definite evidence of over intervention. The natural birth movement was a reaction to that, and like all extreme debates, it's become very very polarized. I think that there is a very polarized debate, and that a lot of people have lost sight of the fact that the only person who matters is the woman. A woman needs knowledge, she needs to be empowered, she needs all the facts, she needs to be supported to make the right decision the right choice for her, her choice is paramount. Whatever that choice is, our job then is to support her, and my frustration is many women are not

being empowered to make the right choice, because they're getting very selective or highly polarized information . . . I feel very sorry for young women, who are coming through the system trying to make this decision, because I wouldn't know where to go to get open, honest, rational advice. You've got OBs [obstetricians] being very defensive and responding badly to accusations of being patriarchal and over interventional. . . . And you've got these absolute zealots on the normal birth side, who are just denying women knowledge, and its anti-feminist . . . It is kind of anti-feminist to lead women up the garden path saying, this is what a perfect birth looks like, and you can do it. And then when they don't do it, and a lot of them don't, they're left high and dry and utterly broken as a result. I think that's one of the most anti-feminist things you can do. So as a result, we need to reclaim the middle ground, and work together to put women back at the center of this debate.

A legal expert provided context for how the medicalization of childbirth was able to silence women's voices: "You know technological and practice advances tend to rapidly outstrip ethical and political advances." Making childbirth a positive experience for women in Ireland requires listening to women and offering woman-centered care that moves beyond a narrow focus on safety while enabling women to take advantage of technology, such as pain relief, through an increase in community-based midwifery care.

TRAVELLER AND ASYLUM-SEEKING WOMEN

Vulnerable and underserved women, including asylum-seeking women and Traveller women, face unique barriers to quality maternity services. Scholars argue that medicalization of perinatal mental health leads to a silencing of women's voices, especially women of color, ethnic minorities, and migrant women.[57] According to the *Confidential Maternal Death Enquiry in Ireland*, out of fifty-four maternal deaths between 2009 and 2018, 30% occurred in women who were not born in Ireland.[58] Furthermore, women born outside of Ireland accounted for 23.4% of all births in Ireland during the same period.[59] As a result, maternal deaths may be over-represented among women born outside of Ireland. According to the 2017 *Perinatal Statistics Report* by the HSE's Healthcare Pricing Office, the stillbirth rate among women from Africa who give birth in Ireland is 6.7%, compared to 3.7% among national Irish women.[60] The early neonatal mortality rate among women from Africa is more than double the rate among national Irish women (3.5% compared to 1.6%), and the perinatal mortality rate (PMR) is almost double (9.8% compared to 5.3%).[61] The chair of AIMS Ireland, Dr. Krysia Lynch said, "These PMR figures are alarming, very disturbing and they need urgent and immediate action . . . For a start, the HSE needs to explain why the mortality rates are higher and what exactly it is doing to reduce them."[62]

Jane X, an activist with MERJ, wrote a blog entry about her experience in a maternity hospital and miscarriage at 22 weeks pregnant. She described her experience as traumatic and cited discrimination, misogyny, and obstetric violence. She wrote: "My main goal is to shed light on what women have been going through in Irish hospitals, particularly women from minority backgrounds whose voices usually go unheard."[63] Patricia Kennedy and Jo Murphy-Lawless have argued in favor of a coherent model of maternity care responsive to the needs of asylum-seeking women, which recognizes their lack of legal support and unique vulnerabilities and offers practical and social support.[64] A recent study of asylum-seeking women's experiences of childbirth in Ireland found a lack of culturally competent care and poor communication with intermittent access to interpreter services.[65] The authors of the study argue that asylum-seeking women have specific needs informed by migratory trauma that complicate their experiences of isolation, vulnerability, and alienation, which are exacerbated by the medicalization of childbirth in Ireland.[66]

The Equal Status Act of 2002 established the Irish Traveller Community as an Indigenous minority group with a distinctive nomadic lifestyle and unique culture, value system, language, and traditions.[67] Compared to the settled population, Travellers have significantly higher fertility, as well as perinatal and infant mortality rates.[68] The 2016 Central Statistics Office found that 31.9% of 15- to 29-year-old Travellers were married, compared with 5.8% of the general population. Nearly half of Traveller women ages 40 to 49 had given birth to five or more children, compared with 4.2% of women overall.[69] The All Ireland Traveller Health Study (AITHS) found that Travellers experience health disparities, including infant mortality, with Traveller infants 3.6 times more likely to die compared with other infants.[70] Overall, the AITHS showed that Travellers face discrimination and experience poor outcomes in health, education, housing, and employment compared to the settled population.[71]

According to Fiona McGaughey, negative and exploitative media coverage of Traveller culture serves to marginalize this community, which already faces exclusion and discrimination in Ireland.[72] These stereotypes influence medical discourse, which ascribes an essentialist view of Traveller women, believing that their cultural beliefs negatively impact pregnancy and childbirth outcomes, which ultimately reifies safety and disempowers women.[73] According to Bernadette Reid and Julie Taylor, Traveller women's attitudes toward pregnancy and childbirth reflect a cultural focus on family and collective identity, with unity and security emphasized through peer support.[74] Given these supportive cultural pillars, "for Traveller women, the negotiation of maternity care seems inconceivable in the absence of practical, emotional and informational support from other women."[75]

Reid and Taylor urge the simplification of application procedures for medical cards, women-held records, and improved record transfer to support nomadism and improve continuity of care.[76]

BREASTFEEDING

Breastival (https://breastival.co.uk/) is an annual festival started in 2017 in Northern Ireland to support and normalize breastfeeding. The goal of the festival is to combat the isolation breastfeeding mothers and families may feel in a culture where breastfeeding is uncommon. Sabina Higgins, wife of Irish President Michael D. Higgins, launched Breastival 2021 with a speech calling for investment in breastfeeding awareness campaigns.[77] Higgins criticized Ireland's breastfeeding rates, with only 45% of women breastfeeding at hospital discharge.[78] Similarly, Ireland's National Women and Infants Health Programme aims to ensure that all maternity services comply with the Baby-Friendly Hospital Initiative (BFHI). The global BFHI recognizes practices that protect and promote breastfeeding, including rooming-in to support mother-newborn bonding. However, according to Abby Bender, "substantive change—not merely higher rates of breastfeeding, but less anxiety, ambivalence, and shame around all feeding practices—requires not only conversations about health and parenting but also an awareness of Irish history and what is buried there."[79] Indeed, breastfeeding as a bodily practice is historical[80] and impacted by the legacy of institutionalization in Ireland. Bender describes the failure of breastfeeding at Mother and Baby Homes, including Bessborough in Cork, where mothers were prevented from breastfeeding or forced to breastfeed under regimented conditions that resulted in insufficient feeding and infant starvation.[81]

Within this context, local and global breastfeeding promotion campaigns perpetuate stigma and aim to control women's bodies.[82]

The unintended consequences of breastfeeding campaigns, such as "Breast Is Best," include a failure to support women's bodily autonomy and cultural preferences. A recent qualitative study of Traveller women found a strong culture of bottle feeding in which women did not feel that they had a choice to breastfeed because of barriers related to shame, embarrassment, and a lack of privacy.[83] The BFHI's majority-norm expectation of breastfeeding and rooming-in is culturally unacceptable for Traveller women.[84] In one study of the maternity needs of asylum-seeking women in Ireland, the vast majority initiated breastfeeding; however, material circumstances did not support continued breastfeeding.[85] According to Bender, "there remains the underlying tension between the professed mission to increase breastfeeding rates and the failure to offer material changes that would make that goal possible for most women, especially those living in direct provision."[86] As with maternity care, women deserve a true choice about whether or not to breastfeed, which requires women-centered care that values women's lived experience and moves beyond a medicalized, essentialist view of breastfeeding to support all of the ways that women choose to nourish their infants.

CONCLUSION

The Bessborough Mother and Baby Home in Cork opened in 1922 and housed 9,768 women and 8,938 children until it closed in 1998. According to the *Final Report of the Commission of Investigation into Mother and Baby Homes*, 923 children died at Bessborough, although only sixty-four burial places were found.[87] By 1934, Bessborough recorded the highest infant mortality rate at a Mother and Baby Home in Ireland. In the late 1940s, Ireland's chief medical officer shut it down for a brief period after 100 out of 180 babies died in one year. The Cork Survivors and Supporters Alliance (CSSA) successfully campaigned to prevent development on the grounds at Bessborough and to memorialize the unknown numbers of women and children who were buried there. In a tweet, the CSSA shared their state-ment: "The mothers wishes are paramount and must be centered in order to avoid re-abuse of their autonomy."[88] In a 2021 interview with BBC, Maureen Considine, a researcher for the CSSA, acknowledged that their success meant that the government "listened to people who historically have not been listened to."[89] The CSSA continues to work toward state-ownership of the burial ground to ensure it is marked and protected into the future.

Improving reproductive experiences in Ireland requires confront-ing the legacy of Mother and Baby Homes and the continued insti-tutionalization of childbirth in hospitals that perpetuates patriarchal and hierarchical control over women's bodies through the medicaliza-tion of childbirth. Medicalization silences women's voices and their lived experiences of childbirth. This struggle will continue to require grassroots organizing and truth-telling to demand change and pre-serve human rights. The need for feminist praxis remains, including the tools the Elephant Collective used to successfully achieve manda-tory inquests for maternal deaths. Making childbirth a positive expe-rience for women in Ireland requires listening to women. Women in Ireland continue to find new ways to use art and technology to raise their voices about their experiences in maternity care. Since 2020, Ireland's *Birth Stories* podcast has shared more than ninety childbirth stories with over 50,000 downloads. Founded by Corah Gernon, a GentleBirth instructor, to provide women an opportunity to share their experiences of pregnancy and childbirth, she wrote: "Sharing your story is not only something to be proud of but it is also giving other women the opportunity to connect with your journey. Hearing their story reflected in yours helps others feel less alone."[90]

Making childbirth a positive experience for all who give birth in Ireland requires offering woman-centered care that moves beyond a narrow focus on safety while enabling women to take advantage of technology, such as pain relief, through community-based midwifery care. In February 2018, the WHO offered new guidelines on intrapartum care and making childbirth a positive experience for women globally.[91] The WHO acknowledges that medicalization of labor and delivery resulting from increased regulation of the physiological process of childbirth may undermine women's ability to give birth. Indeed, the WHO and the UN Global Strategy for Women's, Children's and Adolescents' Health urge medical providers to adopt a woman-centered and human-rights approach to ensure not only that women survive childbirth but also that they achieve a positive experience of childbirth that allows them to thrive. These recommendations emphasize the psychological and emotional needs of women, which includes their right to have control over childbirth through shared decision-making.

In 2019, Ireland's Department of Health established a Women's Health Taskforce to improve women's experiences of healthcare and health outcomes. In the face of recent maternity scandals, the Taskforce aimed to give more consistent, expert, and committed attention to women's health issues. Its initial priority areas include improving gynecological health, supports for menopause, physical activity, and mental health. Specifically, the Taskforce seeks to normalize conversation about women's health through radical listening to hear from women across the lifespan, including minority and disadvantaged women. In March 2022, the Minister of Health launched the Women's Health Action Plan 2022–2023, created by the Taskforce. The action plan includes a new framework for women's health guided by three principles, including listening to women, investing in women's health initiatives, and delivering women's priorities for their health.[92] A reproductive justice approach that privileges the voices of vulnerable and underserved women, including asylum-seeking and Traveller women, is essential to improve quality maternity services. This chapter highlights the continued need for truth-telling to center women's lived experiences in order to disrupt the nature/technology dualism and reconceptualize the essentialist, medicalized process of childbirth to support women's choices in maternity care.

Obstetric Violence

Symphysiotomies and Hysterectomies

In the late 1990s and early 2000s, troubling reports emerged from midwives working inside the Irish maternity care system as well as from women who claimed to have been harmed before, during, or after giving birth in Irish hospitals. First, in the late 1990s, midwives exposed the practices of Dr. Michael Neary of Our Lady of Lourdes Hospital in Drogheda; Neary, they revealed, performed unnecessary hysterectomies on dozens of women in the previous decades. Then, several years later, survivors of symphysiotomy and pubiotomy[1]— outdated procedures performed during obstructed births that had long been replaced elsewhere by the cesarean section—came forward to expose the reality that as many as 1,500 Irish women from the 1940s through 1980s were subjected to these procedures without their consent or, sometimes, even knowledge. Many suffered debilitating physical and emotional effects for years after.[2] Pubiotomy survivor Rita McCann later described her experience: "I was pulled to the bottom of the bed. My legs were strapped into stirrups. I was nine months pregnant, flat on my back . . . I was helpless and I did not know what was going to happen. [Then] I got a local anesthetic and the torture began." McCann also talked about the "agony, literally agony" that she felt during the procedure.[3] By coming forward

Catching Fire. Beth Sundstrom and Cara Delay, Oxford University Press. © Oxford University Press 2023.
DOI: 10.1093/oso/9780197743942.003.0007

and sharing their stories, women like McCann helped to expose an endemic system of obstetric violence that flourished in Irish hospitals for decades.

This chapter examines the hospital-based practices of symphysiotomy and forced hysterectomies in the twentieth century, interpreting them as episodes of obstetric violence and human rights violations. These practices, we argue, provide evidence of the power of physicians and reveal the ways in which religious, national, and biomedical power has been mapped on Irish women's reproductive bodies for decades. The chapter argues that in order to achieve reproductive justice in Ireland, we must confront obstetric violence by foregrounding the experiences, stories, and words of the survivors of these procedures, as well as the activists who helped bring obstetric violence to the public's attention and who continue to work tirelessly to bring a form of justice to survivors.

This chapter also assesses contemporary debates about redress schemes and other forms of reparations that the state has explored or implemented for survivors of obstetric violence. We conclude this analysis with a discussion of justice, asking how victims and survivors of symphysiotomies and hysterectomies can receive justice from a state that is still, at times, unwilling to listen to women's stories and truths and how relevant the transitional justice model is for historical examples of obstetric violence.

OBSTETRIC VIOLENCE AND REPRODUCTIVE JUSTICE

To date, most research on motherhood and women's bodies in modern Ireland has explored the ways in which the bodies of "outcast" women, notably unmarried pregnant women or mothers, were contained and mistreated within Irish institutions. Through the 1990s,

Magdalene laundries, Mother and Baby Homes, schools, prisons, lunatic asylums, and reformatories isolated the bodies of sexually "deviant" women, keeping the rest of Ireland's women and, thus, the nation pure.[4] The abuse of women's bodies within these punitive institutions is well known.[5] Research on how medical, religious, and political systems controlled the bodies of married women who did not enter institutions, however, remains rare. Indeed, forced hysterectomies and symphysiotomies have received less attention than abuses in institutions, in part because their survivors tend to be women who, through marriage and reproduction, conformed somewhat to the ideal of Irish womanhood and, therefore, were not necessarily recognized as obvious and visible victims of what Caelinn Hogan calls the "shame-industrial complex."[6] This reality, and the fact that much media reporting on reproduction in Ireland in recent decades has been on abortion, means that women's experiences of obstetric violence remain somewhat obscure.

Women's health advocates and activists, however, have consistently worked to create a more comprehensive reproductive justice movement in Ireland that moves beyond the most well-known contexts of abortion and institutionalization. As one activist we interviewed articulated:

> I identify as an activist, or identify more with the rally for reproductive rights because for me it was never just about abortion, it was about any form of control of women, control of their bodies, control of their reproductive lives, stuff related to pregnancy, childbirth, to me that's all one argument, it's not just about termination, I suppose with the term bodily autonomy you could get into a whole philosophical argument about what that means but for me it's about bodily integrity, power, domination, oppression of people through their reproductive function and there's a whole history in Ireland of coercion, incarceration

of pregnant women, symphysiotomy scandal, all of these things tie into it. Reproductive justice is more like everything, because I suppose . . . acknowledgement of history, being aware of the fact that women have, for so long, suffered so much at the hand of the state, of the church, and it has been through their function of child bearers and mothers, predominately in my opinion.

This activist's placing of symphysiotomy in conversation with institutional harms and reproductive rights is significant, serving as a call to action for others to consider the regulation of women's bodies in Ireland from a broader, reproductive justice perspective. Another activist we interviewed agreed:

There were a number of things, we had a lot of controversies about reproductive health that weren't specifically linked to the abortion issue, but were culturally linked. . . . we could point to some historic scandals that have happened in Irish maternity hospitals, and the symphysiotomy issues and all those kind of reproductive justice issues were there in the background, I can't remember the consultant who was removing women's wombs unnecessarily, but I remember at the time that was a big issue. Kind of broadening out the abortion issue into decision making.

As these women articulate, broadening our understanding of the harms that the Church-state consensus, in conjunction with the medical profession, enacted on reproductive bodies is an essential step in achieving reproductive justice through truth-telling.

Throughout the twentieth century, it was not only unmarried mothers who had the potential to disrupt Irishness; all parturient women and women of childbearing age were surveilled, monitored, and constructed as passive subjects within the biomedical model of healthcare. Here, again, Ireland's history, placed within a comparative context, is noteworthy. By the nineteenth and twentieth centuries in Europe and the United States, the medical establishment had asserted its power over health and illness through the medicalization of the body.[7] This biomedical power constructed bodies as objects detached from humanity—as machines. For women, this process was more pronounced, resulting in their alienation from not only their bodies but also science and medicine more broadly.[8]

Emily Martin has explored the ways that "science" has been falsely constructed as standing in opposition to "culture." According to Martin, "Although we tend to think of science as outside culture because it seeks the truth about nature, I assert that it is in fact more like a hegemonic system."[9] This means that science is far from an impartial path to absolute truth but rather is as embedded in culture—patriarchy, religion, morality, and so on—as any other human-created system. The lines between science and culture, then, overlap; science and technology are part and parcel of cultural systems. In the cases of forced hysterectomies and symphysiotomy, discussed in detail here, science and, specifically, obstetric practice were determined not by evidence or best practice but by cultural norms and the mores of the hegemonic Church-state system that dominated twentieth-century Ireland.

Recent studies of the Irish healthcare system have underscored its limits and harms, demonstrating how a hybrid mix of public and private services that are grounded in a neoliberal perspective leave behind the most vulnerable and glorify the power of the male physician.[10] Also receiving criticism is the reality that many public hospitals have been or still are managed by religious orders, which has prevented patients from receiving adequate contraception and abortion services, among other things.[11] Catholic religious orders first began managing hospitals in Ireland in the early nineteenth century. By the latter decades of that century, women religious were the majority of Ireland's nurses, and the Sisters of Mercy and other orders dominated hospital-based healthcare, so much so that by independence, "religious involvement and management of health services was well established."[12]

Meanwhile, many politicians and healthcare professionals approached their work with a Catholic ethos, protesting developments or changes in healthcare that challenged Catholic teachings or Church influence. From independence through the 1950s, demographic concerns about high rates of emigration and high infant and child mortality rates resulted in pro-natalist policies but also led to a showdown between some medical professionals and Church leaders. The Mother-and-Child scheme in the early 1950s, which proposed to extend free healthcare services to mothers and families in order to combat infant mortality, became a moment of contention when Catholic leaders, including Dublin's Archbishop McCabe, protested what they viewed as the state's encroachment on its sacred territories: motherhood and family life. When the scheme failed because the government ultimately refused to push it through, effectively bowing to Church authorities, McCabe wrote to colleagues in Rome:

> That the clash should have come in this particular form and under this Government, with Mr Costello at its head, is a very happy success for the Church. The decision of the Government has thrown back Socialism and Communism for a very long time. No Government, for years to come, unless it is frankly Communist, can afford to disregard the moral teaching of the Bishops.[13]

This was a significant moment in the state's history, affirming that the Church would continue to be the dominant power regulating family life. The implications for reproduction were substantial: the failure of the scheme ensured that the state would be reluctant to question the Church's influence on maternity care and that the power of physicians and hospitals would only increase. Writing of the Our Lady of Lourdes Hospital, where Dr. Michael Neary performed unnecessary forced hysterectomies through the 1990s, Sheila O'Connor points out: "Throughout its history, the structure of the maternity hospital was rigidly hierarchical and authoritarian, with either the consultants [physicians] or management of the Medical Missionaries occupying the pivotal position."[14]

In the second half of the twentieth century, forced hysterectomies and symphysiotomies—forms of obstetric violence—proved the veracity of this. Obstetric violence is a useful framework in understanding the harms and human rights violations that biomedical power can impose. In 2014, the World Health Organization (WHO) recognized the abuse and disrespect experienced by women in healthcare facilities globally during labor and delivery. The WHO acknowledged the prevalent practices of verbal and physical abuse, violations of privacy and confidentiality, humiliation and coercion, and unconsented medical procedures, framing them within a human rights context:

> Many women across the globe experience disrespectful, abusive or neglectful treatment during childbirth in facilities. This constitutes a violation of trust between women and their health-care providers and can also be a powerful disincentive for women to seek and use maternal health care services. While disrespectful and abusive treatment of women may occur throughout pregnancy, childbirth and the postpartum period, women are particularly vulnerable during childbirth. Such practices may have direct adverse consequences for both the mother and infant.[15]

According to Michelle Sadler and colleagues, increased medical interventions combined with the abuse and disrespect of women during childbirth have resulted in obstetric violence.[16] This, we contend, is also true for historical examples such as symphysiotomy and forced hysterectomies, which certainly were part and parcel of medicalization and neoliberalism but also derived from pervasive and persistent religious worldviews and, indeed, the conflation of all of these patriarchal forces. In twentieth-century Ireland, an institutionalized, medicalized model combined with unique religious and cultural realities to present an extreme example of obstetric violence, resulting in thousands of women who consequently were disempowered during childbirth.

Carlos Herrera Vacaflor defines obstetric violence as "the violence exercised by health personnel on the body and reproductive processes of pregnant women, as expressed through dehumanizing treatment, medicalization abuse, and the conversion of natural processes of reproduction into pathological ones."[17] Farah Diaz-Tello argues that obstetric violence consists of the "bullying and coercion of pregnant women during birth by health care personnel."[18] The term thus refers to the treatment that people who can become pregnant receive during and after pregnancy from healthcare institutions and experts; it usually occurs during facility-based births and can reference either physical or psychological violence. First articulated by researchers working on twentieth-century Latin America, primarily Venezuela, Brazil, and Mexico in the early 2000s,[19] the term has, in recent years, been utilized by scholars and healthcare professionals across the United States, Australia, and parts of Africa to describe a largely recent phenomenon, with a focus on unnecessary or forced medical interventions, including episiotomies and cesarean sections. In addition to labor and delivery, women may experience obstetric violence during abortion, contraception, prenatal, and postpartum care.[20]

The global reproductive justice community has an important role to play in ending obstetric violence as a human rights violation and ensuring respectful healthcare.[21] It must approach these issues from an intersectional perspective. Women experience mistreatment during childbirth based on a variety of intersecting characteristics, including race/ethnicity, socioeconomic status, education, religion, age, medical conditions, ability, and immigration status.[22] Conversely, women may experience higher quality care when they meet certain ideal characteristics, such as being an adult, white, married, middle class, healthy, completing more education, or carrying an intended pregnancy, among others.[23] In Ireland, motherhood is viewed as a moral status, in which being married offers legitimacy while unmarried women may be condemned.[24] Married women, however, have faced obstetric violence in Ireland as a direct result of the unique combination of the biomedical paradigm and Ireland's restrictive Catholic culture, both of which harnessed women into roles as bearers of multiple children, thus limiting their choice and autonomy and diminishing their whole personhood.

Most analyses of obstetric violence posit that medicalized approaches to childbirth decrease women's rights and autonomy.[25] Moreover, some studies of Latin America and Africa categorize the medicalization of birth and, thus, obstetric violence as colonial or Western interventions.[26] This argument also is relevant in respect to Ireland, a country having a complicated colonial relationship with Great Britain and where medical modernization similarly came at the hands of the imperial state. Ireland's postcolonial culture is also evidenced by the reality that, through 2019, when abortion in Ireland was still criminalized, thousands of Irish women every year accessed it legally through travel to Britain. Ireland, therefore, continued to embody the child-like role of the colonized, exporting its problems to the colonizer.[27]

In twentieth-century Irish history, however, the use of symphysiotomy was not simply a colonial or postcolonial intervention. Instead, it represented a complex response to the legacy of colonialism: while the former colonizer, Britain, adopted advanced medical technology (including cesarean sections) and secular worldviews, Ireland combatted its colonial history by privileging cultural and religious approaches to childbirth and maternal fertility. Contradictory views emerged in Ireland, where because of its association with the former colonizer, medicalized childbirth was somewhat suspect yet impossible to ignore completely. A hybrid system, in which the medical system was intertwined with culture and, specifically, with Catholicism, emerged.

Understanding obstetric violence using a reproductive justice lens considers the historical, social, political, biological, and economic contexts that contribute to inequities based on race/ethnicity, ability, class, sexuality, religion, and immigrant status, among other characteristics. The WHO has urged scholars to investigate, advocate, and engage in dialogue about this critical public health issue. So far, however, most researchers have failed to examine obstetric violence within a historical context. Similarly, Irish Studies scholars have been slow to connect the concept to reproduction in Ireland. It is our contention that the label should be applied to Ireland, both today and throughout its twentieth-century history.[28] Indeed, we argue that Ireland offers a case study of not only the realities of obstetric violence for women but also the effects of it on a nation, and on a postcolonial nation specifically, even decades later.

Moreover, obstetric violence forces us to recognize that the institutionalization of violence against Irish women, usually discussed in reference to what James Smith calls Ireland's institutional "architecture of containment,"[29] extended to, and continues to extend to, the medical sphere. Alongside asylums and schools, hospitals were and are sites of violence against women. Analyzing obstetric violence alongside reproductive justice places Ireland's relationship with reproduction in a historical and comparative context even as it endeavors to privilege the long-overlooked experiences and voices of women themselves.

THE HYSTERECTOMY SCANDAL

In the early 2000s, Dr. Michael Neary, an obstetrician-gynecologist at Our Lady of Lourdes Hospital in Drogheda, was removed from the Irish medical register after giving unnecessary hysterectomies to dozens of women.[30] Several years earlier, two Irish midwives reported that Neary was conducting an unusually high number of cesarean hysterectomies in the hospital.[31] A subsequent government inquiry was established "to determine how many peripartum hysterectomies were carried out in the Maternity Unit from the 1960s onwards and to inquire how these operations were recorded and reviewed."[32] "Out of 39 cases reviewed," the inquiry ultimately "found that 18 represented unacceptable practice, 5 were doubtful and in 16 cases his practice was acceptable." The resulting report also specified that from 1986 to 1998, "ten women had complained about Dr. Neary, claiming to have received unnecessary hysterectomies."[33]

In most of the documented cases, Neary, a respected obstetrician-gynecologist, diagnosed pregnant or birthing patients with rare conditions, including placenta accreta or excessive hemorrhage.[34] When these patients went in for scheduled or emergency cesarean sections, Neary then removed their uteruses and/or ovaries, telling them later that he had done so to save their lives. According to midwives' and birthing women's later testimonies, Neary told his patients that their condition presented a rare, "one-in-a-million" situation that left him no choice but to perform emergency hysterectomies. In some cases, women were not told about their hysterectomies until much later, and for those who were informed before or during the procedure, their consent was not sought or even considered. And it is now clear that most of the hysterectomies that Neary performed were not necessary.

The case of twenty-year-old Niamh, who was a patient of Neary in the late 1990s, is revealing. Dr. Neary actually was the doctor who had assisted at Niamh's birth decades earlier, and Niamh and her family therefore knew and trusted him. After having a seemingly normal cesarean delivery of her first child at the hands of Neary, Niamh later recalled, he told her "he would have to take out my womb. I asked what he was talking about. He said he could not stop the bleeding... If he didn't take it out I would be dead quite soon."[35] Later examinations revealed that there was nothing abnormal about Niamh's birth; the "emergency" hysterectomy was completely unnecessary.

Róisín, another of Neary's patients, was given a hysterectomy after her second child was born via cesarean section. Róisín later remembered that after her child was born, Neary told her that her "womb was not contracting." Before Róisín had time to react, Neary and the rest of the medical staff quickly began the hysterectomy procedure; Róisín's consent was not sought or given. After it was over, a midwife told Róisín that Dr. Neary had acted to "save her life." The subsequent investigation of Neary discovered, however, that Róisín's hysterectomy, like Niamh's, was medically unnecessary and dangerous.[36]

In the 1990s, when several midwives and patients began to complain about Neary, the hospital leadership, and Neary himself, refused to take such complaints seriously. Only after several years, and with the consistent efforts of midwives at the hospital, did an investigation come about. Even then, Irish physicians who were asked to weigh in on the case initially supported Neary; it was only when, at the urging of midwives, non-Irish medical professionals were brought in to examine the evidence that the true picture was revealed. The truth-telling actions of the midwives who reported Neary, and of the women survivors who subsequently came forward, exposed a shocking pattern of obstetric violence and human rights violations at one of Ireland's most respected Catholic maternity hospitals.

The hysterectomy scandal appears at first glance to trouble the ideals of the Irish state—Neary, rather than upholding the goal of fecundity, took away women's abilities to reproduce. We argue, however, that the underlying culture that allowed Neary to commit harms on women's bodies, undetected, for decades is the same as that which allowed symphysiotomy and the criminalization of abortion. The Neary scandal in particular underscored the authority of male physicians and the refusal of many in the maternity-care system to listen to women's voices, validate their experiences, or take the opinions of midwives seriously. Neary's practice at Our Lady of Lourdes Hospital brought to light the collusions between some healthcare practitioners, Church authorities, and state officials that, in turn, revealed, as the official inquiry into the Neary case summarized, "a story set in a time of unquestioning submission to authority": that of the male doctor, the Catholic Church, and the state.[37]

The roles played by midwives in the Neary case shed light on how many obstacles these women had to confront to be heard. In the Irish medical system, midwives and nurses had, since the first few decades of the twentieth century, clearly been taught to obey male physicians under all circumstances. The archives of *An Bord Altranais* (ABA)—the Irish Nursing and Midwifery Board—reveal the pervasiveness of this hierarchy. Starting in the beginning of the twentieth century, the colonial state created new training systems and oversight commissions that nurses and midwives had to work within. After independence in 1922, the new Irish state followed suit. Under the guise of professionalism and hygiene, women carers and healers now had to register with the state, be trained through an approved hospital, wear a uniform, ensure that their tools and midwifery bags were neat and clean, and keep detailed notes on their patients. The eradication of traditional carers, known as "handy-women" in Ireland, was also part and parcel of reform efforts.[38] In 1927, a Local Government Board official read a letter to ABA staff that stated the following:

That no unregistered person shall attend women in childbirth otherwise than under the direction and in the presence of a registered medical practitioner.

That any unqualified person rendering assistance to a woman in childbirth in a case of emergency shall without delay summon a qualified medical practitioner or a midwife to the case.[39]

Those bodies that oversaw medical care were absolutely clear that nurses and midwives were to perform only their duties and defer to the authority of physicians in all circumstances. Midwives were obliged to report to authorities on almost every aspect related to their practices. The Central Midwives Board, Rule E.12 A, for example, stated: "A midwife must notify the Local Supervising Authority of each case in which she has advised the substitution of artificial feeding for breast feeding."[40] The regulation and surveillance of midwives, and their clear subordination within Ireland's medical system, meant that those midwives who initially reported Neary's harmful practices were dismissed, and many more were fearful to come forward.

While it may be tempting to dismiss the forced hysterectomy scandal as the product of one "bad apple," power-hungry physician, the case is revelatory of the larger misogynistic systems deeply entrenched in Ireland that allowed Neary to exercise power and violence while being publicly lauded as a skilled doctor. Neary enacted his violence on women across decades because the Catholic-informed biomedical system not only allowed him to do so but provided a context in which he could flourish. As Rosemary Mander and Jo Murphy-Lawless explain, Neary's power must be contextualized:

[S]uch an assumption of power may begin benignly, even altruistically. But such individuals may develop tunnel vision and become blinkered so that, *in the absence of any opposition,* their conviction of their own rightness and that they have the only answer passes and escalates unchallenged. These increasingly powerful individuals are then positioned to redefine the situation or territory to their own advantage. This effectively disempowers any potential opposition because the powerful individuals are able to present themselves as the solution, albeit to a problem which may not have existed before they created it.[41]

In the case of forced hysterectomies, Neary was empowered by a healthcare system that encouraged physicians to exercise their power indiscriminately. Neary's confidence and public acclaim—created by the medical system and Church-state regime—helped to silence those who may have witnessed his transgressions. Over time, Neary even may have convinced himself that the violent procedures he performed were necessary—the "solution" to a problem that did not exist until he created it.

The government report summarizing the Neary scandal often reads as an apology for Neary and Our Lady of Lourdes. Discussing the hysterectomies that Neary performed during and after cesarean sections, it states:

> In modern obstetrics, such a patient would probably be advised to have a tubal ligation to protect against further pregnancy and the couple would be fully advised to use additional barrier methods of contraception to ensure minimal risk until the effectiveness of the tubal ligation was assured. Male vasectomy might also be discussed as an option. These options were not available at The International Missionary Training Hospital of Our Lady of Lourdes in Drogheda. No forms of contraception advice, apart from the rhythm or Billings method, were countenanced by the

ethos of the owners of the hospital. The obstetricians there, in common with obstetricians in other Catholic hospitals with a Catholic ethos, may have carried out hysterectomies to protect the woman's health from a further pregnancy.[42]

The state's report attempts to provide a rationale for Neary's actions by explicating the hospital's anti-contraception ethos, rather than recognizing that *both* of these things—forced hysterectomies and the prohibition on contraception at hospitals run by religious orders—are part and parcel of the same maternity system that permits, or even encourages, physicians to view women's bodies as objects and deny them reproductive decision-making. What happened at Our Lady of Lourdes in the 1980s and 1990s demonstrates, as Joan McCarthy, Sharon Murphy, and Mark Loughrey write, "the excess of epistemic (knowledge based) and moral authority invested in doctors and clergy, and the correlated lack of such authority invested in midwives and women patients."[43]

The view that Neary was simply a rogue doctor also is challenged by research that has demonstrated an overall high rate of hysterectomies amongst Irish women, particularly young women, beyond the Lourdes Hospital case.[44] To date, this reality has not been explained. Arguments that the hysterectomy scandal at Our Lady of Lourdes was an isolated incident that can be explained by the actions of one deviant doctor lose validity even more when forced hysterectomies are considered alongside other examples of obstetric violence, most notably symphysiotomy. Although the two practices may, at first glance, appear to be strange companions, with symphysiotomy designed ultimately to protect women's fertility and hysterectomy, of course, designed to restrict fertility, both are evidence of the medical system's control of women's bodies.

SYMPHYSIOTOMY

Rosaleen O'Connor was one of hundreds, and possibly thousands, of Irish women who survived symphysiotomies from the 1940s to the 1980s. She later revealed:

> They just took me into the ward and put me on the bed and told me they were going to do some little job . . . "you'll be very sore, and your legs will be tied together," [said the doctor]. And by God, it's a thing you'll never forget the rest of your life.[45]

With the goal of assisting in obstructed births, this outmoded medical practice expands the pelvis through the cutting of surrounding cartilage and ligaments. Abandoned in favor of cesarean sections by the early twentieth century in most places, symphysiotomy persisted in Ireland into the second half of the twentieth century because Catholic doctors there viewed it as less harmful to women's fertility than cesarean sections. Symphysiotomy has been associated with long-term detrimental physical and emotional effects in women.[46] Indeed, in the years and then decades after their symphysiotomies, Irish women survivors endured chronic health problems, including back pain, difficulty walking and lifting things, and incontinence.[47]

Symphysiotomy predated cesarean sections by more than a century. The first successful symphysiotomy in Ireland was completed by W. J. Smyly in the Rotunda Hospital in 1782. Although a handywoman reportedly performed the earliest effective cesarean section in Ireland in Armagh in 1738, it was not until 1890 that Irish physicians could claim a successful outcome with the operation.[48] As cesarean sections grew safer in the early twentieth century, symphysiotomies outside of Ireland became rare; in 1908, Robert Jardine, Professor of Midwifery in Glasgow, reflected contemporary medical opinion when he argued that he was not "very much in favour" of symphysiotomies because they offered greater "risk[s] to the child" than the increasingly preferred cesarean section.[49] By the 1940s, the availability and efficacy of antibiotics transformed the practice of cesarean section; in the United States and Britain in particular, the use of cesarean sections in obstructed births increased rapidly throughout the twentieth century.[50] Meanwhile, in Europe and the United States, symphysiotomy had been abandoned as a viable medical procedure by the middle of the century.

Things were different, however, in independent Ireland. The state's overtly Catholic worldview complicated the practice of cesarean sections, which were thought at the time to be tantamount to contraception—popular medical opinion asserted that a woman could only undergo three cesarean sections in a lifetime before sterilization would become necessary. Vehemently opposed to any limitation to women's childbearing capabilities, some Irish political, religious, and medical authorities viewed the cesarean section as an untenable option. Alex Spain, Master of Dublin's National Maternity Hospital, argued in 1948 that although he believed cesarean sections were fundamentally safe, he did not see them becoming accepted in Ireland due to cultural rather than medical forces. "It will, however, be a long time before such a method of delivery will be easily accepted by the profession or by the community at large," he wrote. "The results will be contraception, the mutilating operation of sterilization and marital difficulty, matters often too lightly considered by the medical profession but of immense importance in any community, especially where the great body or any large number of the people subscribe to the Catholic rule."[51]

Oonagh Walsh, author of the 2014 government-sponsored report on symphysiotomy, affirms that the main proponents of symphysiotomy, Alex Spain and Arthur Barry of Ireland's National Maternity Hospital, "were both devout Catholics, serving a predominantly Catholic patient population, and they made no secret of their willing conformity to religious precepts in the treatment of patients."[52] While most of their peers in Europe and the United States had discounted symphysiotomy, some Irish physicians preferred its use in challenging deliveries, ostensibly so that married Irish women could continue to bear children without any impediments. In symphysiotomy cases, then, religious and cultural norms, rather than evidence or best medical practice, affected physicians' decisions and, as a result, determined women's reproductive experiences. The example of symphysiotomy in Ireland reminds us that the relationship between "science," "technology," and "culture" is complex and frequently convoluted.

In 1944, the National Maternity Hospital, Dublin, followed soon by the Coombe Maternity Hospital, began to choose symphysiotomy as the best option in the case of an obstructed birth. Overall, approximately twenty-four Irish hospitals performed the procedure throughout the mid to late twentieth century, after it already had been abandoned in most other places.[53] Notably, however, not all Irish maternity hospitals followed suit. According to Jacqueline Morrissey, doctors at the Rotunda—Ireland's oldest lying-in hospital—did not favor symphysiotomies and pubiotomies by the mid-twentieth century and, indeed, criticized their use in Ireland.[54] This reality provides further evidence that some Irish medical institutions ignored debates about best medical practice in favor of supporting the Catholic ethos of the state—blurring the lines between "science" and "culture."

Some survivors of symphysiotomy maintain that the Catholic ethos of the state and women's patriotic responsibilities to bear children for Ireland were explicitly discussed by doctors and nurses preparing women for the procedure. According to Rosemary, for example, who survived the procedure in Dublin in 1957, the conversation with her physician went as follows: "You're a Catholic family, De Valera[55] said, you'd be expected to have at least ten [children]. I normally do a Caesarean section, but because you are such a good Catholic, I'll do a symphysiotomy, I'd no idea what it was. I'll have to stretch your hips and straighten your pelvis, he said."[56] By referencing the staunchly Catholic De Valera, architect of the constitution's assertion that women were primarily mothers, Rosemary's physician privileged the religious ethos of the new state over best and accepted medical practice. The 2012 Halappanavar case and recent debates about abortion testify that this blueprint of allowing culture, not science, to inform reproductive decision-making has continued into contemporary Ireland, exposing a persistent and insidious pattern.[57]

According to symphysiotomy researcher Marie O'Connor, as many as 1,500 women received symphysiotomies and pubiotomies in Ireland from the 1940s through the 1980s; by 2011, she maintains, only between 150 and 200 survivors were left alive in the country.[58] The claims of some of these surviving women have exposed the link between symphysiotomy and obstetric violence. These women contend that they not only suffered pain and infirmity from the procedure later in life but also were coerced into symphysiotomies and, in some cases, never even told at the time that their pelvises had been separated during birth. Some studies have "found that degrading treatment and loss of dignity and control during birth can contribute to birth trauma and even postpartum post-traumatic stress disorder."[59] The effects of obstetric violence on women, then, include not only pain, disability, humiliation, and shame, but also post-traumatic stress disorder.[60]

Overall, an examination of symphysiotomy testifies to the importance of interrogating coercion and consent, bodily autonomy and violence, and cultural power in Irish culture. It also provides historical context for the contemporary debates in Ireland surrounding women's reproductive rights, as well as for scholars seeking to analyze reproductive justice in Ireland. Activists we interviewed explicitly recognized these connections, encouraging us not to focus on abortion to the exclusion of other topics such as symphysiotomy:

Savita Halappanavar's story isn't about refusing an abortion, it's a story about interpreting the law to require this really cruel treatment . . . as well similarly it is about positively saying the law requires me as a Catholic doctor, an observant doctor, whatever . . . mental health, and physical health can possibly sustain. So I think by leaving symphysiotomy out of the story, we're really missing the point I suppose and that's why symphysiotomy means a lot to me, if that makes sense. There's a lot there.

Several women who were given symphysiotomies in twentieth-century Ireland maintain that they did not consent to having the procedures done, and many did not even know that they had endured a symphysiotomy or pubiotomy until well after the fact.[61] Suffering in later years from pain and disability, some of these women sought answers, often across decades, yet continued to be rebuffed by medical authorities. According to one survivor: "I had to go to the doctor, it was a few years after. The doctor didn't tell me what was wrong with me, no one did. He didn't examine me, no one did."[62] Another recalled: "I just remember being brought into a theatre and the place was packed with people. I wasn't told what was happening . . . I was screaming and being restrained. I couldn't see much except for them sawing. It was excruciating pain . . . I was just 27 and I was butchered."[63] Kathleen of Cork later claimed that during her 1957 symphysiotomy,

> the sister tutor had written "query [Caesarean] section?" on my notes. Over my dead body, said [Dr] Sutton. . . . They didn't tell me what they were doing. I thought I had paralysis. I couldn't move my legs up or down . . . I asked what was wrong; nobody told me. It was a case of shut up. You felt you were up against a brick wall . . . I can't make out why they didn't section me . . . He [Sutton] cracked it [the pubic bone].[64]

The ways in which doctors and nurses treated pregnant women's bodies loom large in women's recollections. According to Vera, who was given a symphysiotomy in Drogheda in 1968:

> He [the doctor] came in with a big entourage. It was very invasive, you were tied up, you had no control. There was a good crowd there, nurses, other people behind him, two or three—other doctors I took them to be—juniors, students . . . My feet were tied up in stirrups for the symphysiotomy, I had gas and air. I must have fainted off, the nurse came with a bowl of water and a facecloth, and splashed water all over my face. These are the things you remember. I hated it, it was not nice, I still don't like it [splashing water on my face]. I was in terrible distress. What he did to me—you have no power, when your legs are caught up like that.[65]

Vera's reminiscences attest that medical staff took control of her body, restraining it and positioning it as they wished, thus denying her bodily autonomy. Like Vera, many women who birthed in Irish hospitals had "no control," "no power" over their reproductive experiences.

According to Sarah Cohen Shabot, the abuse and dominance of the maternal body through obstetric violence in patriarchal societies "appears to be necessary in order to domesticate these bodies, to make them 'feminine' again." The bodies of laboring women, she argues, are naturally "healthy" and "powerful." They thus contest the myth of passive femininity and must be brought back in control by means of restraint and violence. It is this, then, that makes obstetric violence explicitly gendered and categorized as violence against women.[66] Symphysiotomy in Ireland should be interpreted as obstetric violence not only because Irish medical professionals restrained the female body during childbirth, rendering it acceptably passive, but also because the procedure caused extensive, and sometimes life-long, pain, disability, and infirmity, thus immobilizing women, or at least hindering their mobility and, thus, their agency, for decades. Similarly, forced hysterectomies removed women's reproductive decision-making capabilities and caused significant emotional distress for some. Both examples reveal "women's bodies as the site of battles waged in relation to sexuality and reproductive autonomy."[67] Even today, when Irish doctors perform unnecessary cesarean sections, they restrain and often paralyze women's bodies, rendering them passive. During cesarean sections, physicians instead take on the role of actor in childbirth, making a clear statement about power and authority.[68] In Ireland, this practice follows historical precedent.

TRUTH-TELLING

"We can be under no illusions," argues legal scholar Joanne Conaghan, "about the extent to which Irish women have suffered as a consequence of State-sanctioned, often religiously fomented misogyny."[69] If forced hysterectomies and symphysiotomy are clear evidence of this misogyny, they also serve as examples of how activists and protestors have worked tirelessly to enact change. Both also are examples of ethical communication and truth-telling.

In the hysterectomy scandal, midwives at Our Lady of Lourdes Hospital doggedly attempted to expose Neary and tell the truth about the procedures he performed on women. Ann, one of the midwives who ultimately exposed Neary's harmful practices, insisted on telling the truth despite the opposition she faced. As the government report into Neary later wrote of Ann:

Her colleagues either did not wish to countenance such criticisms, or found reasons to disprove her perceptions . . . Her colleagues told her that she had no evidence so she had taken to carefully documenting what she saw in theatre . . . She was told however that there was nothing anyone could do unless a patient actually complained.[70]

Survivors of forced hysterectomies at Lourdes Hospital also pushed for an official inquiry of Neary. Once news about the scandal began to trickle out in the late 1990s and early 2000s, they organized themselves into a group called "Patient Focus" and publicly demanded a government investigation. They met with each other and created support groups. Individually and collectively, they also told their story to the Irish public. One survivor, Catriona Molloy, shared her experience on a popular radio show in 2006, saying:

> I myself didn't feel as if I was in a life or death situation because I was really angry with the way I had been treated in the hospital that day. I was giving out stink about the way I felt neglected the whole day in the hospital . . . nobody really seemed to be listening to me . . . I felt like a piece of meat on a slab . . . it was like you were on a conveyer belt, just another person passing through, it [birth] wasn't a memorable occasion.[71]

Like those women who told their truths about abortion travel, Molloy and other survivors of Neary gave voice to their bodily experiences as well as the lack of autonomy and control they faced. In 2007, the Irish government agreed to spend 45 million euros to compensate the survivors of forced hysterectomies at Our Lady of Lourdes. A total of 172 women were deemed eligible to receive reparations.[72]

Kept secret through most of the twentieth century, the reality of Ireland's symphysiotomy history only became apparent as the new millennium approached. In 1999, after the *Irish Times* published an article on symphysiotomy by Dr. Jacqueline Morrissey, who was researching the practice, Ireland's Institute of Obstetricians and Gynaecologists responded by defending the practice.[73] This in turn prompted survivors of the procedure to organize. In 2002, Survivors of Symphysiotomy (SOS) came into being; it continues, today, to advocate for the women who endured these operations. SOS's messages have challenged the notion that symphysiotomies were sometimes necessary and perhaps the result of only a few incompetent physicians. Rather, as Máiréad Enright explains, SOS has consistently underscored the culture that underpinned the medical system, exposing the reality that "Catholic activist doctors, working in hospitals that pursued a Catholic ethos, revived and developed symphysiotomy in the 1940s in an attempt to adapt medical practice to Catholic reproductive imperatives."[74]

The membership of SOS is significant because it challenges the assumption that activism is the realm of the young. In 2002, SOS was created by symphysiotomy survivor Mathilda Behan, who was then in her 70s, and led by other mature women survivors. Protesting in front of the Irish Parliament and publicizing their message via Facebook, these survivor-activists claimed physical and digital space. They publicly shamed the government into confronting symphysiotomy and recognizing their personal experiences. When the Irish government was slow to respond, SOS also took their case to the United Nations to force the state to conduct a fair and impartial inquiry into symphysiotomy.[75]

Still, survivors remain dissatisfied and disappointed in the government's response. In 2016, the government finally published a report on symphysiotomy—the Walsh Report—that laid out a redress or payment scheme for survivors but, in the view of SOS, did not adequately explore the pervasiveness of the procedure or recognize its effects on survivors. In this report, the government recognized almost 400 women as being entitled to redress as survivors of symphysiotomy.[76] The payment scheme provided for the following:

Category 1A: symphysiotomy only €50,000
Category 1B: symphysiotomy with significant disability as
defined in the Scheme €100,000
Category 1C: a particular form of symphysiotomy, with or
without significant disability €100,000–€150,000

SOS responded with criticisms, writing that "the price that comes
with a survivor taking the comparatively small compensation is that
they must also waive their right to seeking a judicial remedy, which is
a right given to us by the United Nations Human Rights Committee.
These failings could constitute as human rights infringements."[77] The
announcement of the redress scheme placed some survivors in a difficult position: the money that the government offered could help
them with their continuing medical bills, but accepting the money
meant that they could make no further claims or pursue other legal
avenues.

In addition, SOS charged that the investigation into symphysiotomy discounted the voices and experiences of survivors. Máiréad
Enright summarizes:

[The report] locates symphysiotomy in the universal, ahistori-
cised progressive time of scientific development; as a necessary
response to religious circumstances since overcome. Walsh is
constructed from a range of historical medical literature and
hospital statistics. It did not examine personal medical records.
It only drew on a small number of survivors' testimony because
members of SOS boycotted the interviews. They did this to
protest a draft report, published in 2012, which established the
report's main conclusions before survivors were consulted.[78]

Claims that the Walsh Report did not adequately consider the experiences and voices of survivors resonate today after the controversial

2021 government-sponsored Mother and Baby Homes report, which has been widely denounced as ignoring, or even suppressing, survivor testimony and stories.[79]

Recent scholarship on the Mother and Baby Homes and Magdalene laundries has grappled extensively with the issue of a governmental response to historical harms, pointing out how, as Katherine O'Donnell, Maeve O'Rourke, and James Smith write, "state-led efforts to address this legacy of abuse have been inadequate, and as a result the harms experienced are not 'historical' but continuing."[80] How can the state best grapple with the harms of both institutions and obstetric violence? One potential answer is to adopt a transitional justice approach that centers truth-telling and women's embodied realities. Scholars and some governments are increasingly recognizing the utility of transitional justice for addressing historical harms beyond war and conflict. Transitional justice

> engages the practice of criminal accountability, including the trials of perpetrators whether by local or international courts, truth commissions, vetting and lustration of state institutions, reparations, acknowledgement, apologies, memorials, exhumations of mass graves, quotas and affirmative action practices, security sector reform and modalities of political accommodation, particularly associated with transitional compacts.[81]

Because it encourages the foregrounding of survivor and victim experiences and voices, transitional justice has proven to be a successful form of truth-telling in various contexts. In Canada, for example, beginning around 2010, the government implemented transitional justice programs to account for the state's historic abuse and institutionalization of Indigenous peoples. Beginning with an exploration of the forcing of Indigenous children into Catholic Indian Residential Schools, Canada's Truth and Reconciliation Commission committed to "learn the truth about what happened in the residential schools and inform all Canadians of these findings."[82] In 2019, Canada's National Inquiry into Missing and Murdered Indigenous Women and Girls (MMIWG) also adopted a transitional justice approach. Significantly, it moved beyond considering the harms of those placed in institutions, addressing the physical and sexual violence that Indigenous women and girls suffered as well as the cultural violence they endured. It recognized these harms as structural and historical, foregrounding not only interpersonal violence but also

> the seizure of traditional lands, expropriation and commercial use of Indigenous cultural objects without permission by indigenous communities, misinterpretation of indigenous histories, mythologies and cultures, suppression of their languages and religions, and even the forcible removal of Indigenous peoples from their families and denial of their indigenous identity.[83]

By acknowledging the links between different forms of oppression, such as cultural violence and physical violence, the MMIWG established a precedent for broadening transitional justice and truth-telling. It also brought to the international public's attention the need to engage in a gendered approach to transitional justice and to showcase the harms suffered by women and girls in misogynistic cultural systems—"to address the sustained, systematic, and deeply wounding human-rights and humanitarian-law violations experienced by women."[84]

Canadian efforts, moreover, have forced a reconsidering of the relationship between colonialism and forms of violence, publicizing the need for a recognition and accounting of colonialism in transitional justice. Bill Rolston and Fionnuala Ní Aoláin make a compelling case for considering colonialism in Ireland when discussing transitional justice and, indeed, argue that a transitional justice process must grapple with the colonialism itself, recognizing the links between colonialism and the harms that the post-colonial state inflicted on its people.[85]

These models are being applied now by scholars working on Ireland. In the Irish context, while transitional justice was first employed as a way to account for the "Troubles"—Northern Ireland's late twentieth-century civil war[86]—advocates, activists, and scholars recently have been applying the concept to the institutions that abused thousands of Irish people: Catholic-run schools, reformatories, Mother and Baby Homes, and Magdalene laundries. That most victims and survivors of these institutions were women and girls has spurred scholarship on the relationship between gender analysis and transitional justice. Fionnuala Ní Aoláin points out that transitional justice has been a "predominantly masculine field," cautioning that we need a rethinking of transitional justice from a gendered perspective. She also argues that in many cases involving women, a narrow focus on rape and sexual violence during conflict has precluded other investigations.[87] We would argue that the expansion of transitional justice to institutions (rather than a narrow focus on war and conflict) is a welcome one, but that it, too, must be broadened in the Irish case to consider obstetric violence.

CONCLUSION

Symphysiotomy and forced hysterectomies may offer the clearest examples of obstetric violence in the Irish context, but they are by no means the only relevant case studies. The treatment of unmarried mothers, and specifically their containment within institutions, including Mother and Baby Homes and Magdalene laundries, forced adoptions, as well as the maternity restrictions imposed during the COVID-19 pandemic, provide further evidence of how the Irish state has enacted violence upon the bodies of reproductive women.[88] The effects of this violence are extensive. Sara Cohen Shabot demonstrates that survivors of obstetric violence face significant long-term effects, including feelings of "embodied oppression, of the diminishment of self, of physical and emotional infantilization."[89] As Orla O'Connor of the National Women's Council of Ireland recently remarked, "One day, Ireland must accept and understand the extent and prevalence of institutional abuse of women and children."[90] Understanding Ireland's complex history of obstetric violence, as well as the potential for reproductive justice to provide solutions for moving forward, are essential in this process. For symphysiotomy and forced hysterectomy survivors, however, who grow older with every passing year and with every new reproductive controversy that erupts in Ireland, that day may come too late.

Conclusion

When Judge Maureen Harding Clark released the Irish government's 2016 report outlining compensation for women who received symphysiotomies, activists described Ireland's maternity services as "an ongoing horror story."[1] In response to this criticism, Irish obstetricians published a letter in *The Irish Times* describing their dedication to providing quality, woman-centered care, despite ongoing challenges.[2] Some healthcare providers started tweeting with the hashtag #WeAreDelivering to demonstrate their commitment to delivering quality healthcare. Some activists countered this message with the trending hashtag #IBirthed to refocus the dialogue on women's autonomy and agency in childbirth. In a blog post, Sinéad O'Rourke of AIMS (Association for Improvements in the Maternity Services) Ireland described the backlash against #WeAreDelivering:

> By repeating the term "delivering," you continue to create an environment in which women cede control of their pregnancies and birth to you, the professionals. Where choices made by women are secondary to the knowledge and expertise of those who treat them.[3]

Catching Fire. Beth Sundstrom and Cara Delay, Oxford University Press. © Oxford University Press 2023. DOI: 10.1093/oso/9780197743942.003.0008

The history and current dialogue surrounding Mother and Baby Homes, symphysiotomy, and other episodes in reproductive health present an opportunity to build a thriving reproductive justice movement in Ireland. According to Leslie Sherlock, "reproductive justice is the intersectional movement that Ireland is ready for, and the time is now."[4]

Truth-telling supports a reproductive justice approach to women's health by motivating institutions to listen to women. Grassroots truth-telling forced improvement and transparency in the CervicalCheck screening program and lead to coalition-building to counteract HPV vaccination misinformation. Through truth-telling, advocates demonstrated that contraceptive access remains one of the most critical issues facing women and convinced the government to budget for free contraception beginning in 2023. The 2018 Repeal movement, which privileged women's stories and social media activism, led to a successful vote overturing the anti-abortion Eighth Amendment to the Irish Constitution. The legacy of the Eighth Amendment offered leverage to reform the National Maternity Strategy and current maternity practices. Feminist praxis by the Elephant Collective successfully demanded mandatory inquests for maternal deaths through the Coroners (Amendment) Act 2019. However, the *In Our Shoes— Covid Pregnancy* social media campaign uncovered gender inequity in government policies during a time of crisis and revealed the continuing need for systemic change to ensure every woman's human right to high-quality, respectful maternity care in all circumstances.

All people have the human right to make autonomous decisions about their own bodies. The future of women's health activism in Ireland demands a reproductive justice approach that privileges the voices of vulnerable and underserved women, including asylum-seeking, ethnic-minority, and Traveller women, as well as trans and gender-expansive people. We have discussed how some critics claim that the Together for Yes campaign for Repeal marginalized diverse voices in favor of a mainstream message. However, activists acknowledged the intersectional nature of the ongoing human rights movements in Ireland, including the overlap between people who campaigned for marriage equality in 2015 and the campaign for Repeal in 2018. According to one activist we interviewed, women's health activism in Ireland is "very much a queer movement":

> The LGBT and queer community were very much a driving force for abortion rights in Ireland, historically and contemporaneously. A more recent and explicit example being the great work done by Radical Queers Resist in blocking the very graphic imagery outside the maternity hospital in Dublin so that people walking in and out wouldn't have to see it.

An intersectional reproductive justice movement was also evident in the ways that activist groups who formed for Repeal continued to work together toward ending Direct Provision, homelessness, and Church control of education.

This book features the understudied voices of women's health activists who have challenged high-tech myth systems to redefine women's health and reproduction, making these central concerns in Irish society and government. This insight contributes to the disruption of the nature/culture dualism and highlights the possibilities of empowerment through technology in women's health.[5] The Irish case offers important insight into understandings of gender, science, and technology in the global movement for women's autonomy. Indeed, Ireland's human rights movements provide evidence for how campaigners may engage with digital intersectional communication to develop transparent and reflexive social media advocacy.[6] We argue that ethical communication is an integral element of reproductive justice, and that truth-telling and digital intersectional communication allowed women's health activists in Ireland to triumph over unethical communication that was grounded in historical and cultural misogyny.

Activists identified Repeal Shield during the Repeal campaign as essential to supporting digital intersectional communication and empowering campaigners. A member of Repeal Shield we interviewed said that "it's an information war" on social media rife with repetitive misinformation, abuse without consequence, and the constant threat of doxing. Activists, then, must "engage at their own peril" on social media. Repeal Shield used technology to counter technology, creating a supportive online environment to facilitate grassroots organizing and truth-telling. One campaigner that we interviewed said about Repeal Shield:

> It infuriated [anti-choice opponents] so much they couldn't get to us, couldn't argue or frighten us. We were just all positive, all the time . . . You fake it until you make it and then you actually end up feeling really empowered. So that's what I learned from social media, no matter what's happening you come out saying "I feel really supported, this is a great campaign" and it was and we did!

Repeal Shield fostered digital intersectional communication by removing the frustration and distraction of trolls and automated bots, which allowed activists to tell stories and engage in conversations with real people.

Technology continues to change women's health activism in Ireland as advocates continue to find new ways to use art and technology to raise the voices of asylum-seeking, ethnic-minority, and Traveller women, as well as trans and gender-expansive people about their experiences in healthcare. In late 2021, TranScribe Health launched a platform for trans people to anonymously and safely share their stories and experiences with healthcare.[7] The story-sharing coalition identified a number of demands, including that the government disband the National Gender Service, which regulates and restricts the healthcare of trans people.

Since 2006, women in Ireland have accessed safe telemedicine abortion through Women on Web.[8] Founded by Dr. Rebecca Gomperts in 2005, Women on Web is a Canadian nonprofit organization that provides telemedicine access to contraception as well as mifepristone and misoprostol in countries without safe termination of pregnancy care.[9] It aims to save women's lives and to help individuals fulfill the World Health Organization's definition of health, which moves beyond the absence of disease to include physical, mental and social well-being. Between 2006 and 2019, when abortion was not yet available in Ireland, Women on Web served more than 10,000 women from Ireland and Northern Ireland. In the second year of legal access to abortion in Ireland, online abortion-seeking from Women on Web decreased. Although Irish abortion services provided needed care for most reasons, women with an abusive partner still preferred to access Women on Web rather than local abortion care.[10] To reduce reliance on international abortion services, Jo Greene and colleagues suggest normalizing abortion care and increasing awareness of care and access pathways, providing free and confidential services, and supporting local telemedicine abortion services, including text-based contact for those with an abusive partner.[11]

In 2018, Dr. Gomperts founded Aid Access to serve women in the United States for the first time.[12] This nonprofit emerged in response to more than a decade of laws and policies progressively restricting and eliminating access to abortion in the United States. State-by-state, forced-birth activists passed targeted regulation of abortion providers (TRAP) laws dictating unreasonable provider qualifications, facility specifications, and reporting requirements. Laws in certain states required parental notification or parental consent. Laws required medically unnecessary waiting periods, which were sometimes linked to biased and inaccurate counseling or forced transvaginal ultrasound. Aid Access was the first online telemedicine service to offer mifepristone and misoprostol to everyone in the United States. Between 2018 and 2020, Aid Access received over 57,000 requests from people in all fifty states.[13] Dr. Gomperts was named one of *Time* Magazine's 100 most influential people of 2020 for providing safe abortion around the world.

On June 24, 2022, the US Supreme Court's decision in *Dobbs v. Jackson Women's Health* overturned *Roe v. Wade*, eliminating the federal constitutional right to abortion. Since then, Aid Access has received approximately 4,000 requests per day, although the need may be greater since social media apps, including Instagram and Facebook, have limited access to information by removing posts about abortion services. The US Constitution is grounded in the right to liberty, which includes the right to make choices about family, relationships, marriage, bodily integrity, medical decision-making, and bodily autonomy. The right to abortion is tied to these other essential liberties.

As the Irish case shows, eliminating the right to abortion far exceeds the restriction of one personal decision, impacting the human right of all people to make autonomous decisions about their body and their life. The current situation in the United States exemplifies how comprehensively fifty years of progress can be dismantled. It also highlights the global need for the reproductive justice movement that Irish activist groups purposively built after Repeal by continuing to work together to improve healthcare and end homelessness, Church control of education, and Direct Provision, among other issues.

Irish activists and abortion-rights advocates responded to the overturning of *Roe* in the summer of 2022 with shock, anger, and resolve. Retired Irish obstetrician-gynecologist and former head of the National Maternity Hospital Dr. Peter Boylan told reporters that

American "women will die as a consequence of this."[14] Labour party leader Ivana Bacik wrote in the *Irish Examiner* that as the United States "steps backwards," the Republic of Ireland must continue to "move forward." Responding to the US Supreme Court's decision, Bacik argued that it "should strengthen [Ireland's] resolve to ensure effective access to safe, legal terminations of pregnancy," but that it also "serves as a powerful reminder to us here in Ireland, and across the world, that we can never take progress on women's rights for granted."[15] Ailbhe Smyth, co-director of Together for Yes during the Repeal campaign, responded to *Dobbs* by articulating worries that this decision will have a "knock on effect," spurring a contraction of abortion rights globally.[16]

Within this global context, Ireland has served as a model for the abortion struggles of other countries. Indeed, grassroots truth-telling has been adopted globally to oppose abortion restrictions. Shortly after Ireland's Repeal campaign, the National Congress in Argentina passed a law in 2020 allowing abortion during the first fourteen weeks of gestation. In September 2021, a referendum to reform an abortion ban in San Marino passed in a popular vote, due to the work of women's health activists. Recently, there have also been positive changes in abortion laws in Mexico, South Korea, and Thailand. Irish campaigners have also supported Poland as a Constitutional Court there further restricted abortion access in 2020, which led to mass protests and the creation of the Abortion Dream Team to resist these human rights violations. In Malta, where abortion is illegal in all circumstances, activists have employed the digital intersectional communication strategies popularized in Ireland. Break the Taboo Malta collected real women's abortion experiences and published their stories anonymously to emphasize that abortion is normal. Malta's "Dear Decision Makers" Campaign aims to change the views of policy-makers by collecting and sharing personal testimonies from women who have been harmed by the abortion ban and healthcare providers who are forced to provide suboptimal care to their patients.

As Maeve Higgins suggests, there is evidence of an "electric" women's health activism in Ireland.[17] Women's health activist movements in Ireland have, indeed, been "catching," reforming CervicalCheck, legalizing abortion, enacting the Coroners (Amendment) Act, and leading the on-going investigation of Mother and Baby Homes. This fire has also been contagious globally, spreading and supporting a human rights reproductive justice approach to gender equity. In the wake of the 2022 overturning of *Roe v. Wade* in the United States, Women on Waves launched a crowdfunding campaign for a new post-*Roe* strategy. Women on Waves, founded by Dr. Gomperts in 1999, provides abortion services on ships and through robots and drones, as well as offering workshops and developing art projects.[18] Its new strategy involves collecting clinical trial data to register mifepristone as a weekly, on-demand contraceptive in order to distribute it as a method of contraception, thereby disrupting the difference between contraception and abortion. They argue that this "game-changing contraceptive strategy" will be enacted by "women—and those who love them—who will make the change."[19]

Activists in Ireland have developed novel ways to employ technology to engage in grassroots truth-telling and digital intersectional communication. In everyday ways, such as developing Repeal Shield to protect and nurture activists, campaigners challenged high-tech myth systems by disrupting the nature/culture dualism. By valuing women's embodied experience, activists reimagined the use of technology, challenging patriarchal norms and empowering women to tell their stories. As abortion rights and reproductive justice movements in the United States and around the globe ignite in the wake of the *Dobbs* decision, these activist strategies—and the broader lessons of the Irish case—are more relevant than ever.

NOTES

Introduction

1 Although abortion was already criminalized under the United Kingdom's 1861 Offences Against the Person Act, in 1983 the Eighth Amendment went further, equating fetal life with the life of a pregnant person: "The State acknowledges the right to life of the unborn and, with due regard to the equal right to life of the mother, guarantees in its laws to respect, and, as far as practicable, by its laws to defend and vindicate that right" (*The Eighth Amendment of the Constitution*, 1983).

2 Maeve Higgins, "What Irish Women Know," *The New York Times*, May 24, 2018, https://www.nytimes.com/2018/05/24/opinion/irish-women-abortion-vote.html.

3 Magdalene laundries and Mother and Baby Homes, managed by orders of the Catholic Church but supported by the Irish state, were used to contain and control housed women (or girls in some cases) suspected of having committed a sexual transgression or to house pregnant unmarried women or mothers and their children, often until the latter were illegally adopted out.

4 Cara Delay and Beth Sundstrom, "The Legacy of Symphysiotomy in Ireland: A Reproductive Justice Approach to Obstetric Violence," in *Reproduction, Health, and Medicine*, vol. 20 (Bingley, UK: Emerald Publishing Limited, 2019), 197–218, https://doi.org/10.1108/S1057-629020190000020017; Paul Michael Garrett, "Excavating the Past: Mother and Baby Homes in the Republic of Ireland," *British Journal of Social Work* 47, no. 2 (March 2017): 358–74,

https://doi.org/10.1093/bjsw/bcv116; Marie O'Connor, *Bodily Harm: Symphysiotomy and Pubiotomy in Ireland, 1944–92* (Cathair na Mart: Evertype, 2011); Jo Murphy-Lawless, "The Silencing of Women in Childbirth or Let's Hear It from Bartholomew and the Boys," *Women's Studies International Forum* 11, no. 4 (1988): 293–98.

5 In this book, we use the words "women" and "people" interchangeably and inclusively to recognize the need by a variety of individuals for reproductive health services regardless of gender identity. Our approach here is informed by the following statement from the National Advocates for Pregnant Women (NAPW): "Historically, the State has targeted people identified as women for discrimination and state control based on pregnancy and their capacity for pregnancy. The overwhelming majority of people NAPW has represented and advocated for have been identified in public records as women. In addition, the research and data available on many of our issues typically employ the word 'women.' NAPW recognizes, however, that not all people with the capacity for pregnancy identify as women and that the gender binary itself contributes to systems of discrimination and control. NAPW's work is intended to contribute to an all-encompassing fight for civil and human rights—in other words, a true personhood movement. To that end, NAPW uses the terms 'women,' 'pregnant people' and 'people with the capacity for pregnancy' in recognition of the fact that all people are entitled to dignity, equality, and fairness regardless of gender identity, capacity for pregnancy, pregnancy, or stage of pregnancy including labor and delivery." https://www.nationaladvocatesforpregnantwomen.org/napws-work/follow-napw/.

6 "Let's Talk Real: The Abortion Referendum," *The Gibraltar Magazine*, May 31, 2021, https://thegibraltarmagazine.com/lets-talk-real-the-abortion-referendum/.

7 Katherine O'Donnell, Maeve O'Rourke, and James M. Smith, "Editors' Introduction: Toward Transitional Justice in Ireland? Addressing Legacies of Harm," *Éire-Ireland* 55, no. 1–2 (2020): 13, https://doi.org/10.1353/eir.2020.0000.

8 Caelainn Hogan, *Republic of Shame: Stories from Ireland's Institutions for "Fallen Women"* (Dublin: Penguin Ireland, 2019); James M. Smith, *Ireland's Magdalen Laundries and the Nation's Architecture of Containment* (South Bend, IN: University of Notre Dame Press, 2007).

9 Claire Bracken and Cara Delay, "Editors' Introduction: Women's Health and Reproductive Justice in Ireland," *Éire-Ireland* 56, no. 3/4 (Fall/Winter 2021): 6.

10 Clara Fischer, "Gender, Nation, and the Politics of Shame: Magdalen Laundries and the Institutionalization of Feminine Transgression in Modern Ireland," *Signs* 41, no. 4 (2016): 822.

11 *Justice for Magdalenes Research*, http://jfmresearch.com/; Orla Lynch, James Windle, and Yasmine Ahmed, *Giving Voice to Diversity in Criminological Research* (Bristol: Bristol University Press, 2021), https://bristoluniversitypress.co.uk/giving-voice-to-diversity-in-criminological-research; O'Donnell, O'Rourke, and Smith, "Editors' Introduction."

12 James Gallen, "Transitional Justice and Ireland's Legacy of Historical Abuse," *Éire-Ireland* 55, no. 1 (2020): 35, https://doi.org/10.1353/eir.2020.0002.

13 Melissa Brown et al., "#SayHerName: A Case Study of Intersectional Social Media Activism," *Ethnic and Racial Studies* 40, no. 11 (September 2, 2017): 1831–46, https://doi.org/10.1080/01419870.2017.1334934.

14 Jennifer Vardeman and Amanda Sebesta, "The Problem of Intersectionality as an Approach to Digital Activism: The Women's March on Washington's Attempt to Unite All Women," *Journal of Public Relations Research* 32, no. 1–2 (March 3, 2020): 7–29, https://doi.org/10.1080/1062726X.2020.1716769.

15 Taryn De Vere, "40pc of Maternal Deaths in Ireland Are Migrant and Ethnic Minority Women," *HerFamily.ie*, https://www.herfamily.ie/pregnancy/40-of-maternal-deaths-in-ireland-are-migrant-women-293482.

16 "#10thdss: Intersectionality and the Irish Abortion Rights Campaign of 2018," *Emma Q Burns* (blog), September 19, 2018, https://emmaqburns.com/2018/09/19/10thdss-intersectionality-and-the-irish-abortion-rights-campaign-of-2018/. See also Deirdre Niamh Duffy, "From Feminist Anarchy to Decolonization: Understanding Abortion Health Activism before and after the Repeal of the 8th Amendment," *Feminist Review* 124, no. 1 (2020): 69–85, https://doi.org/10.1177/0141778919895498.

17 Katie Mishler, "'It's Most Peculiar that This Particular Story Doesn't Get Told': A Reproductive-Justice Analysis of Storytelling in the Repeal Campaign in Ireland, 2012–18," *Éire-Ireland* 56, no. 3/4 (Fall/Winter 2021): 86.

18 *MERJ: Migrants and Ethnic-minorities for Reproductive Justice*, accessed December 14, 2021, https://merjireland.org/.

19 Fiona de Londras, "'A Hope Raised and Then Defeated'? The Continuing Harms of Irish Abortion Law," *Feminist Review* 124, no. 1 (2020): 44, https://doi.org/10.1177/0141778919897582; Houses of the Oireachtas, "Health (Regulation of Termination of Pregnancy) Act 2018—No. 31 of 2018—Houses of the Oireachtas," text, September 27, 2018, Ireland, https://www.oireachtas.ie/en/bills/bill/2018/105.

20 Bridget E. Keown, "'There Is No Limit to What Could Be Done': Considering the Past and Potential of Irish Queer Health Activism," *Éire-Ireland* 56, no. 3/4 (Fall/Winter 2021): 213.

21 Camilla Fitzsimons, Ruth Coppinger, and Sinéad Kennedy, *Repealed: Ireland's Unfinished Fight for Reproductive Rights* (London: Pluto Press, 2021), 11.

22 J. W. Creswell, *Research Design: Qualitative, Quantitative, and Mixed Methods Approaches*, 4th ed. (Thousand Oaks, CA: Sage Publications, 2014).

23 Rodney G. S. Carter, "Of Things Said and Unsaid: Power, Archival Silences, and Power in Silence," *Archivaria* 61 (September 25, 2006): 215–33; Marika Cifor and Stacy Wood, "Critical Feminism in the Archives," *Journal of Critical Library and Information Studies* 1, no. 2 (May 3, 2017), https://doi.org/10.24242/jclis.v1i2.27; Nydia A. Swaby and Chandra Frank, "Archival Experiments, Notes and (Dis)Orientations," *Feminist Review* 125, no. 1 (2020): 4–16, https://doi.org/10.1177/0141778920931874.

24 Swaby and Frank, "Archival Experiments," 9.

25 Bracken and Delay, "Editors' Introduction," 10.

26 Patricia Hill Collins and Silma Birge, *Intersectionality* (New York: Polity Press, 2016).

27 Joyce M. Nielsen, *Feminist Research Methods: Exemplary Readings in the Social Sciences* (New York: Routledge, 2019).

28 Sharlene Hesse-Biber, *Feminist Research Practice: A Primer,* 2nd ed. (Thousand Oaks, CA: Sage, 2014).

29 Jennifer Aengst and Linda L. Layne, "The Need to Bleed? A Feminist Technology Assessment of Menstrual-Suppressing Birth Control Pills," in *Women, Science, and Technology: A Reader in Feminist Science Studies,* ed. Mary Wyer, Mary Barbercheck, Donna Cookmeyer, Hatice Ozturk, and Marta Wayne (New York: Routledge, 2014), 171–92, citing Donna Haraway, "Situated Knowledges: The Science Question in Feminism and the Privilege of Partial Perspective," *Feminist Studies* 14(3), 1988: 575–599.

30 Jutta Weber, "From Science and Technology to Feminist Technoscience," in *Women, Science, and Technology: A Reader in Feminist Science Studies,* ed. Mary Wyer, Mary Barbercheck, Donna Cookmeyer, Hatice Ozturk, and Marta Wayne (New York: Routledge, 2014), 543–71.

31 Hesse-Biber, *Feminist Research Practice.*

32 Gayle Letherby, *Feminist Research in Theory and Practice* (New York: McGraw-Hill International, 2003).

33 Shulamit Reinharz, *Feminist Methods in Social Research* (New York: Oxford University Press, 1992).

34 United Nations, *International Conference on Population and Development Programme of Action* (New York: United Nations Population Fund, 1994), https://www.unfpa.org/publications/international-conference-population-and-development-programme-action.

35 Kimala Price, "What Is Reproductive Justice? How Women of Color Activists Are Redefining the Pro-Choice Paradigm," *Meridians* 10, no. 2 (2010): 42–65, https://doi.org/10.2979/meridians.2010.10.2.42; Loretta Ross, *Radical Reproductive Justice: Foundation, Theory, Practice, Critique,* vol. First Feminist Press edition (New York: The Feminist Press at CUNY, 2017); Loretta Ross and Rickie Solinger, *Reproductive Justice: An Introduction* (Oakland: University of California Press, 2017).

36 SisterSong, "Reproductive Justice," *SisterSong.net*, accessed December 14, 2021, https://www.sistersong.net/reproductive-justice.

37 Ross and Solinger, *Reproductive Justice.*

38 Price, "What Is Reproductive Justice?"

39 Jo Murphy-Lawless, "Holding the State to Account: 'Picking Up the Threads' for Women Who Have Died in Irish Maternity Services," *Éire-Ireland* 56, no. 3/4 (Fall/Winter 2021): 51–79.

40 Tanya Saroj Bakhru, "Reproductive Health and Human Rights: Lessons from Ireland," *Journal of International Women's Studies* 18, no. 2 (January 31, 2017): 27–29.

41 Murphy-Lawless, "Holding the State to Account," 55.

42 "Applicant C" was part of the A, B, and C v. Ireland case in 2009. See Katherine Side, "A Geopolitics of Migrant Women, Mobility, and Abortion Access in the Republic of Ireland," *Gender, Place & Culture: A Journal of Feminist Geography* 23, no. 12 (2016): 1788–1799.

43 Aoife Bhreatnach, *Becoming Conspicuous: Irish Travellers, Society and the State, 1922–70* (Dublin: University College Dublin Press, 2006).

44 Bernadette Reid and Julie Taylor, "A Feminist Exploration of Traveller Women's Experiences of Maternity Care in the Republic of Ireland," *Midwifery* 23, no. 3 (2007): 249.

45 Clara Fischer, "Abortion and Reproduction in Ireland: Shame, Nation-Building and the Affective Politics of Place," *Feminist Review* 122, no. 1 (2019): 33, https://doi.org/10.1177/0141778919850003.

46 Ciara Breathnach, "Handywomen and Birthing in Rural Ireland, 1851–1955," *Gender & History* 28, no. 1 (April 2016): 34–56, https://doi.org/10.1111/1468-0424.12176.

47 Caitriona Clear, *Women of the House: Women's Household Work in Ireland, 1922–1961* (Dublin: Irish Academic Press, 2000), 99.

48 Don O'Leary, *Biomedical Controversies in Catholic Ireland* (Cork: Eryn Press, 2020).

49 O'Leary, *Biomedical Controversies.*

50 Laura Kelly, "Debates on Family Planning and the Contraceptive Pill in the Irish Magazine Woman's Way, 1963–1973," *Women's History Review* 30, no. 6 (October 29, 2020): 203, https://doi.org/10.1080/09612025.2020.1833495, citing Monica McEnroy, "The Contraceptive Pill in Ireland: Personal Involvement," *Woman's Way*, September 23, 1966.

51 Fitzsimons, Coppinger, and Kennedy, *Repealed*, 7; Hogan, *Republic of Shame.*

52 "Canada," *International Center for Transitional Justice*, https://www.ictj.org/our-work/regions-and-countries/canada.

53 O'Donnell, O'Rourke, and Smith, "Editors' Introduction."

54 Hala Bassel, "Acts of Truth Telling and Testimony in the Conceptualization of Reparations in Post-Conflict Peru," *Global Society* 34, no. 1 (January 2,

2020): 84–98, https://doi.org/10.1080/13600826.2019.1668360; Alison Crosby and M. Brinton Lykes, "Mayan Women Survivors Speak: The Gendered Relations of Truth Telling in Postwar Guatemala," *International Journal of Transitional Justice* 5, no. 3 (November 1, 2011): 456–76, https://doi.org/10.1093/ijtj/ijr017; Margaret Urban Walker, "Truth Telling as Reparations," *Metaphilosophy* 41, no. 4 (2010): 525–45, https://doi.org/10.1111/j.1467-9973.2010.01650.x.

55 Emily Rosser, "The Messy Practice of Building Women's Human Rights: Truth-Telling and Sexual Violence in Guatemala," *Latin American Policy* 6, no. 1 (2015): 68–88, https://doi.org/10.1111/lamp.12061.

56 Bassel, "Acts of Truth Telling and Testimony."

57 Walker, "Truth Telling as Reparations."

58 Karen Brounéus, "Truth-Telling as Talking Cure? Insecurity and Retraumatization in the Rwandan Gacaca Courts," *Security Dialogue* 39, no. 1 (March 1, 2008): 55–76, https://doi.org/10.1177/0967010607086823.

59 Gallen, "Transitional Justice and Ireland's Legacy," 38.

60 Crosby and Lykes, "Mayan Women Survivors Speak."

61 Leigh Gilmore, "He Said/She Said: Truth-Telling and #MeToo," *FORUM: University of Edinburgh Postgraduate Journal of Culture & the Arts*, no. 25 (December 18, 2017): 2–3, http://www.forumjournal.org/article/view/2559.

62 Jasmine R. Linabary, Danielle J. Corple, and Cheryl Cooky, "Feminist Activism in Digital Space: Postfeminist Contradictions in #WhyIStayed," *New Media & Society* 22, no. 10 (October 1, 2020): 1827–48, https://doi.org/10.1177/1461444819884635; Hester Baer, "Redoing Feminism: Digital Activism, Body Politics, and Neoliberalism," *Feminist Media Studies* 16, no. 1 (January 2, 2016): 17–34, https://doi.org/10.1080/14680777.2015.1093070; Kaitlynn Mendes, Jessica Ringrose, and Jessalynn Keller, *Digital Feminist Activism: Girls and Women Fight Back Against Rape Culture* (Oxford: Oxford University Press, 2019).

63 Barbara Sharf and M. L. Vanderford, "Illness Narratives and Social Construction of Health," in *Handbook of Health Communication*, ed. Theresa L. Thompson and Nancy Grant Harrington (New York: Routledge, 2008), 9–34; Beth Sundstrom, "Mothers 'Google It Up:' Extending Communication Channel Behavior in Diffusion of Innovations Theory," *Health Communication* 31, no. 1 (January 2016): 91–101, https://doi.org/10.1080/10410236.2014.936339.

64 Mendes, Ringrose, and Keller, *Digital Feminist Activism*, 16.

65 Thomas K. Houston et al., "The Art and Science of Patient Storytelling—Harnessing Narrative Communication for Behavioral Interventions: The ACCE Project," *Journal of Health Communication* 16, no. 7 (August 2011): 686–97, https://doi.org/10.1080/10810730.2011.551997.

66 Sonja Vivienne and Jean Burgess, "The Digital Storyteller's Stage: Queer Everyday Activists Negotiating Privacy and Publicness," *Journal of Broadcasting*

& Electronic Media 56, no. 3 (July 2012): 362–77, https://doi.org/10.1080/08838151.2012.705194.

67 Zakiya Luna, *Reproductive Rights as Human Rights: Women of Color and the Fight for Reproductive Justice* (New York: NYU Press, 2020), 164.

Chapter 1

1 Gabriel Scally, "Scoping Inquiry into the CervicalCheck Screening Program" (Dublin: Department of Health, 2018), https://www.gov.ie/en/publication/aa6159-dr-gabriel-scallys-scoping-inquiry-into-cervicalcheck/.

2 Beth Sundstrom et al., "A Reproductive Justice Approach to Understanding Women's Experiences with HPV and Cervical Cancer Prevention," *Social Science & Medicine* 232 (July 1, 2019): 289–97, https://doi.org/10.1016/j.socscimed.2019.05.010.

3 Andrew Tinker, "Communication Ethics and the Rejection of Paternalism in John Stuart Mill's *On Liberty*," *Communication Quarterly* 67, no. 3 (May 27, 2019): 312–32, https://doi.org/10.1080/01463373.2019.1596140.

4 Annette M. Holba, "Review of Dialogic Ethics," *Language and Dialogue* 8, no. 3 (2018): 490.

5 Jennifer Vardeman and Amanda Sebesta, "The Problem of Intersectionality as an Approach to Digital Activism: The Women's March on Washington's Attempt to Unite All Women," *Journal of Public Relations Research* 32, no. 1–2 (March 3, 2020): 24, https://doi.org/10.1080/1062726X.2020.1716769.

6 Vardeman and Sebesta, "The Problem of Intersectionality."

7 Anja Nyberg, "Achieving Reproductive Justice: Some Implications of Race for Abortion Activism in Northern Ireland," *Feminist Review* 124, no. 1 (2020): 165–72, https://doi.org/10.1177/0141778919894912.

8 Health Service Executive (HSE), "Cervical cancer," https://www2.hse.ie/conditions/cervical-cancer/overview/.

9 HSE, "Cervical cancer."

10 Kate T. Simms et al., "Impact of Scaled up Human Papillomavirus Vaccination and Cervical Screening and the Potential for Global Elimination of Cervical Cancer in 181 Countries, 2020–99: A Modelling Study," *The Lancet Oncology* 20, no. 3 (March 1, 2019): 394–407, https://doi.org/10.1016/S1470-2045(18)30836-2.

11 "Human Papillomavirus (HPV) and Cervical Cancer," *World Health Organization*, February 22, 2022, https://www.who.int/en/news-room/fact-sheets/detail/human-papillomavirus-(hpv)-and-cervical-cancer.

12 Scally, "Scoping Inquiry."

13 Kate T. Simms et al., "Impact of HPV Vaccine Hesitancy on Cervical Cancer in Japan: A Modelling Study," *The Lancet Public Health* 5, no. 4 (April 1, 2020): e223–34, https://doi.org/10.1016/S2468-2667(20)30010-4.

14 US Food and Drug Administration (FDA), "Gardasil 9," *FDA.gov*, December 10, 2014, https://www.fda.gov/vaccines-blood-biologics/vaccines/gardasil-9.

15 Global Advisory Committee on Vaccine Safety (GACVS), "Safety Update of HPV Vaccines," *Weekly Epidemiological Record* 92, no. 2 (2017): 13–20.

16 "Ten Threats to Global Health in 2019," *World Health Organization*, https://www.who.int/news-room/spotlight/ten-threats-to-global-health-in-2019.

17 Global Advisory Committee on Vaccine Safety (GACVS), "Communication about the Safety of Human Papillomavirus Vaccines," *Weekly Epidemiological Record* 94, no. 51/52 (2019): 613–28.

18 Zakiya Luna, *Reproductive Rights as Human Rights: Women of Color and the Fight for Reproductive Justice* (New York: NYU Press, 2020), 213.

19 G. Spray, *Blood, Sweat & Tears: The Hepatitis C Scandal* (Dublin: Wolfhound Press, 1998).

20 Kimala Price, "What Is Reproductive Justice? How Women of Color Activists Are Redefining the Pro-Choice Paradigm," *Meridians: Feminism, Race, Transnationalism* 10, no. 2 (2010): 42–65.

21 Dionne P. Stephens, Vrushali Patil, and Tami L. Thomas, "STI Prevention and Control for Women: A Reproductive Justice Approach to Understanding Global Women's Experiences," in *Reproductive Justice: A Global Concern*, ed. Joan C. Chrisler (Santa Barbara, CA: Praeger, 2012), 117–44; Sundstrom et al., "A Reproductive Justice Approach."

22 P. De and H. Budhwani, "Human Papillomavirus (HPV) Vaccine Initiation in Minority Americans," *Public Health* 144 (March 1, 2017): 86–91, https://doi.org/10.1016/j.puhe.2016.11.005; Amy M. Burdette et al., "Race-Specific Trends in HPV Vaccinations and Provider Recommendations: Persistent Disparities or Social Progress?," *Public Health* 142 (January 1, 2017): 167–76, https://doi.org/10.1016/j.puhe.2016.07.009; Sharon M. Bond et al., "Racial and Ethnic Group Knowledge, Perceptions and Behaviors about Human Papillomavirus, Human Papillomavirus Vaccination, and Cervical Cancer among Adolescent Females," *Journal of Pediatric and Adolescent Gynecology* 29, no. 5 (October 1, 2016): 429–35, https://doi.org/10.1016/j.jpag.2016.02.005.

23 Bernadette Reid and Julie Taylor, "A Feminist Exploration of Traveller Women's Experiences of Maternity Care in the Republic of Ireland," *Midwifery* 23, no. 3 (September 1, 2007): 248–59, https://doi.org/10.1016/j.midw.2006.03.011.

24 Judith Bush, "'It's Just Part of Being a Woman': Cervical Screening, the Body and Femininity," *Social Science & Medicine* 50, no. 3 (February 1, 2000): 429–44, https://doi.org/10.1016/S0277-9536(99)00316-0.

25 Sundstrom et al., "A Reproductive Justice Approach."

26 Alison Crosby and M. Brinton Lykes, "Mayan Women Survivors Speak: The Gendered Relations of Truth Telling in Postwar Guatemala," *International Journal of Transitional Justice* 5, no. 3 (November 1, 2011): 456–76, https://doi.org/10.1093/ijtj/ijr017.

27 Leigh Gilmore, "He Said/She Said: Truth-Telling and #MeToo," *FORUM: University of Edinburgh Postgraduate Journal of Culture & the Arts*, no. 25 (December 18, 2017), http://www.forumjournal.org/article/view/2559.

28 Sonja Vivienne and Jean Burgess, "The Digital Storyteller's Stage: Queer Everyday Activists Negotiating Privacy and Publicness," *Journal of Broadcasting & Electronic Media* 56, no. 3 (July 2012): 362–77, https://doi.org/10.1080/08838151.2012.705194.

29 Daniel DiMaio, "Nuns, Warts, Viruses, and Cancer," *Yale Journal of Biology and Medicine* 88, no. 2 (2015): 127.

30 Scally, "Scoping Inquiry."

31 Clara Fischer, "Gender and the Politics of Shame: A Twenty-First-Century Feminist Shame Theory," *Hypatia* 33, no. 3 (2018): 371.

32 *Migrants and Ethnic-minorities for Reproductive Justice (MERJ)*, April 29, 2019, https://merjireland.org/index.php/2019/04/.

33 *Migrants and Ethnic-minorities for Reproductive Justice (MERJ)*, April 27, 2018. https://www.facebook.com/MERJIreland/posts/pfbid02rzAtNxvf5MH-Zu3hdeBTZRZRjpiUomcTP7Ve9fy61AN7j2d47xUx6NjkeJzPXDeXvl

34 Ronald C. Arnett and François Cooren, *Dialogic Ethics* (Amsterdam/Philadelphia: John Benjamins Publishing Company, 2018).

35 Liz Farsaci, "Increase in Abuse on CervicalCheck Staff; Delays & Anxiety Caused 'Perfect Storm,'" *Daily Mirror*, December 6, 2019, https://www.pressreader.com/ireland/irish-daily-mirror/20191206/281814285735928.

36 Brendan O'Shea, "Patients—and Medics—Need to See a Quick and Honest Response when Things Go Seriously Wrong," *Irish Independent*, December 4, 2019.

37 Aine McMahon, "Women and Families Affected by CervicalCheck Hail Apology as 'Watershed Moment,'" *Press Association Newswire*, October 22, 2019.

38 Leo Varadkar, "Taoiseach's CervicalCheck Apology in Full," *RTE NEWS*, October 22, 2019.

39 McMahon, "Women and Families Affected by CervicalCheck."

40 "Simon Harris: CervicalCheck Staff 'Subjected to Abuse,'" *Irish Examiner*, December 6, 2019.

41 Fischer, "Gender and the Politics of Shame," 839.

42 Emily Rosser, "The Messy Practice of Building Women's Human Rights: Truth-telling and Sexual Violence in Guatemala," *Latin American Policy* 6, no. 1 (2015): 68–88, https://doi.org/10.1111/lamp.12061; Margaret Urban Walker, "Truth Telling as Reparations," *Metaphilosophy* 41, no. 4 (2010): 525–45, https://doi.org/10.1111/j.1467-9973.2010.01650.x.

43 Rosser, "The Messy Practice."
44 Gilmore, "He Said/She Said."
45 Rosser, "The Messy Practice."
46 McMahon, "Women and Families Affected by CervicalCheck."
47 Daniel Artus, Heidi Larson, and Patty Kostkova, "Role of Social Media in Vaccination Debate about HPV: The VAC Medi+Board Study," *European Journal of Public Health* 29, no. Supplement 4 (November 1, 2019): ckz185.682, https://doi.org/10.1093/eurpub/ckz185.682; Simms et al., "Impact of HPV Vaccine Hesitancy."
48 Gregory D. Zimet and Nosayaba Osazuwa-Peters, "There's Much Yet to Be Done: Diverse Perspectives on HPV Vaccination," *Human Vaccines & Immunotherapeutics* 15, no. 7–8 (August 3, 2019): 1459, https://doi.org/10.1080/21645515.2019.1640559.
49 Sharon J. B. Hanley et al., "HPV Vaccination Crisis in Japan," *The Lancet* 385, no. 9987 (June 27, 2015): 2571, https://doi.org/10.1016/S0140-6736(15)61152-7.
50 David Robert Grimes, "Terminally Ill at 25 and Fighting Fake News on Vaccines," *The New York Times*, December 11, 2019, https://www.nytimes.com/2019/12/11/opinion/anti-vaccine-HPV.html.
51 Simms et al., "Impact of HPV Vaccine Hesitancy."
52 Grimes, "Terminally Ill at 25."
53 Gabe Mythen and Mads P. Sørensen, "Unscrambling Risk, Contesting Expertise: The Case of the Human Papillomavirus (HPV) Vaccine," in *Ageing, the Body and the Gender Regime,* ed. Jude Robinson and Susan Pickard (New York: Routledge, 2019), 38–52.
54 Sundstrom et al., "A Reproductive Justice Approach."
55 Grimes, "Terminally Ill at 25."
56 Mythen and Sørensen, "Unscrambling Risk, Contesting Expertise."
57 Brenda Corcoran, Anna Clarke, and Tom Barrett, "Rapid Response to HPV Vaccination Crisis in Ireland," *The Lancet* 391, no. 10135 (May 26, 2018): 2103, https://doi.org/10.1016/S0140-6736(18)30854-7.
58 Artus, Larson, and Kostkova, "Role of Social Media in Vaccination Debate."
59 Simms et al., "Impact of HPV Vaccine Hesitancy," e232.
60 Jamie Horder, "Toll of Vaccine Hesitancy," *Nature Human Behaviour* 4 (2020): 335; Simms et al., "Impact of HPV Vaccine Hesitancy."
61 Hugo Aznar and Marcia Castillo-Martin, "'Vulnerability' as the Key Concept of a Communicative Ethics for the 21st Century," *Media Development* 4 (2018): 18.
62 Aznar and Castillo-Martin, "'Vulnerability' as the Key Concept," 19.
63 Artus, Larson, and Kostkova, "Role of Social Media in Vaccination Debate."
64 HSE Ireland, "Our Health Service: Meet Laura Brennan," https://www.hse.ie/eng/about/our-health-service/making-it-better/meet-laura-brennan.html.

65 Vicky Phelan (@PhelanVicky), Twitter, May 10, 2018.https://twitter.com/PhelanVicky/status/99449819698140364.8.

66 Grimes, "Terminally Ill at 25."

67 Laura Brennan, *Don't Be Swayed by Rumors* (Dublin: Health Service Executive, 2018), https://www.youtube.com/watch?v=Mw9bkA2eRvI.

68 Mythen and Sørensen, "Unscrambling Risk, Contesting Expertise."

69 Aznar and Castillo-Martin, "'Vulnerability' as the Key Concept," 19.

70 Luis Saboga-Nunes and Patty Kostkova, "Online Anti-Vaccination Movements: The Role of Social Media in Public Health Communications," *European Journal of Public Health* 29, no. 4 (November 1, 2019): 250.

71 Kara Fox, "A Scandal over Cervical Checks Is a Sign of a Bigger Problem in Ireland," *CNN*, accessed January 29, 2022, https://www.cnn.com/2019/10/05/europe/ireland-cervical-check-scandal-intl/index.html.

72 Brian MacCraith, "Independent Rapid Review of Specific Issues in the CervicalCheck Screening Programme" (Dublin: Health Service Executive, 2019), https://www.hse.ie/eng/services/news/media/pressrel/hse-statement-in-response-to-the-maccraith-review.html.

73 Vicky Phelan (@PhelanVicky), Twitter, August 8, 2019. https://twitter.com/PhelanVicky/status/1159623537474396161.

74 Fox, "A Scandal over Cervical Checks."

75 Aznar and Castillo-Martin, "'Vulnerability' as the Key Concept," 19.

76 Crosby and Lykes, "Mayan Women Survivors Speak."

Chapter 2

1 HSE Ireland, "Free Contraception Contract Scheme," https://www.hse.ie/eng/about/who/gmscontracts/free-contraception-service-contract/.

2 Government of Ireland, "Report of the Working Group on Access to Contraception," October 2019, https://assets.gov.ie/38063/89059243e7504 15ebf7e96247a4225ae.pdf.

3 Caroline O'Doherty, "Birth Control Use Here among EU Lowest," *Irish Examiner*, November 18, 2014, https://www.irishexaminer.com/news/arid-20298253.html.

4 Erin Darcy, *In Her Shoes: Women of the Eighth* (New Island, 2020); "In Her Shoes—Women of the Eighth," https://www.facebook.com/InHerIrishSh oes/. See also Cara Delay and Beth Sundstrom, "'In Her Shoes' and in Her Words: Voices, Silences, and Bodies in Irish Women's Abortion Narratives," *Frontiers: A Journal of Women Studies* 43, no. 2 (2022): 139–68.

5 Ashling Bourke et al., "Factors Associated with Crisis Pregnancies in Ireland: Findings from Three Nationally Representative Sexual Health Surveys,"

Reproductive Health 12, no. 1 (March 2, 2015): 2, https://doi.org/10.1186/s12 978-015-0005-z.

6 Bourke et al., "Factors Associated with Crisis Pregnancies," 9.

7 Cliodhna Russell, "One Third of Irish Women Don't Use Contraception," *TheJournal.ie,* February 7, 2014, https://www.thejournal.ie/one-third-irish-women-dont-use-contraception-1319331-Feb2014/.

8 Alison Begas, "New Research Shows Majority of Women in Ireland Are Using Ineffective Contraception to Prevent Pregnancy," *Dublin Well Woman Centre* (blog), November 24, 2020, https://wellwomancentre.ie/new-research-shows-majority-of-women-in-ireland-are-using-ineffective-contraception-to-prevent-pregnancy/.

9 *In Her Shoes,* January 27, 2018, https://www.facebook.com/InHerIrishShoes/photos/a.142385323102560/144962656178160.

10 Tom Inglis, "Origins and Legacies of Irish Prudery: Sexuality and Social Control in Modern Ireland," *Éire-Ireland* 40, no. 2 (2005): 9, https://doi.org/10.1353/eir.2005.0022.

11 Orla McBride, Karen Morgan, and Hannah McGee, *Irish Contraception and Crisis Pregnancy Study 2010 (ICCP-2010): A Survey of the General Population* (Dublin: Health Service Executive Crisis Pregnancy Programme, 2012), 22, https://doi.org/10.25419/rcsi.10770506.v2.

12 Government of Ireland, "Report of the Working Group on Access to Contraception," 15.

13 *In Her Shoes,* June 9, 2018. https://www.facebook.com/InHerIrishShoes/photos/a.142348133106279/170240266983732.

14 Clara Fischer, "Abortion and Reproduction in Ireland: Shame, Nation-Building and the Affective Politics of Place," *Feminist Review* 122, no. 1 (2019): 822, https://doi.org/10.1177/0141778919850003.

15 Lindsey Earner-Byrne and Diane Urquhart, *The Irish Abortion Journey, 1920–2018* (New York: Palgrave Macmillan, 2019); Fischer, "Abortion and Reproduction in Ireland"; Paul Michael Garrett, "Excavating the Past: Mother and Baby Homes in the Republic of Ireland," *British Journal of Social Work* 47, no. 2 (March 2017): 358–74, https://doi.org/10.1093/bjsw/bcv116; Brian Girvin, "An Irish Solution to an Irish Problem: Catholicism, Contraception and Change, 1922–1979," *Contemporary European History* 27, no. 1 (February 2018): 1–22, https://doi.org/10.1017/S0960777317000443; Agata Ignaciuk and Laura Kelly, "Contraception and Catholicism in the Twentieth Century: Transnational Perspectives on Expert, Activist and Intimate Practices," *Medical History* 64, no. 2 (2020): 163–72, https://doi.org/10.1017/mdh.2020.1; Jennifer Redmond, "'Sinful Singleness'? Exploring the Discourses on Irish Single Women's Emigration to England, 1922–1948," *Women's History Review* 17, no. 3 (2008): 455–76, https://doi.org/10.1080/09612020801924597; Jennifer Redmond, *Moving Histories: Irish Women's Emigration to Britain*

from Independence to Republic (Liverpool: University Press, 2018); James M. Smith, *Ireland's Magdalen Laundries and the Nation's Architecture of Containment* (South Bend, IN: University of Notre Dame Press, 2007).

16 Bourke et al., "Factors Associated with Crisis Pregnancies," 8.

17 Ronit Lentin, "(M)Other Ireland: Migrant Women Subverting the Racial State?," in *Race and Immigration in the New Ireland*, ed. Heather Ireland, Julieann Veronica Ulin, and Sean T. O'Brien (Notre Dame, IN: University of Notre Dame Press, 2013), 51–74.

18 Katherine Side, "The Effects of 'Geographies of Accommodation' on Sexual and Reproductive Healthcare: Asylum Seekers in Ireland," unpublished paper.

19 "Research with Young Migrant Women on Sex, Fertility and Motherhood," *sexualwellbeing.ie*, April 2014, https://www.sexualwellbeing.ie/for-professionals/research/research-summaries/research-with-young-migrant-women-2014.pdf.

20 "Research with Young Migrant Women."

21 Catherine Conlon, Joan O'Connor, and Siobhán Ní Chatháin, *Attitudes to Fertility, Sexual Health and Motherhood amongst a Sample of Non-Irish National Minority Ethnic Women Living in Ireland* (Dublin: Health Service Executive, 2012), 107.

22 Conlon, O'Connor, and Ní Chatháin, *Attitudes to Fertility*, 13.

23 Conlon, O'Connor, and Ní Chatháin, *Attitudes to Fertility*, 15.

24 "Our Work," AkiDwA (blog), accessed January 12, 2022, https://akidwa.ie/our-work/.

25 Irish Family Planning Association, "Irish Family Planning Association Submission on Direct Provision to the Oireachtas Committee on Justice and Equality," May 2019, 2–3, https://www.ifpa.ie/app/uploads/2019/06/Direct-Provision.pdf.

26 Bernadette Reid and Julie Taylor, "A Feminist Exploration of Traveller Women's Experiences of Maternity Care in the Republic of Ireland," *Midwifery* 23, no. 3 (September 2007): 248, https://doi.org/10.1016/j.midw.2006.03.011.

27 Pavee Point, "Our Geels: All Ireland Traveller Health Study Pavee Point," 2003, 75, https://www.ucd.ie/t4cms/AITHS_SUMMARY.pdf.

28 Reid and Taylor, "A Feminist Exploration of Traveller Women's Experiences," 252.

29 Reid and Taylor, "A Feminist Exploration of Traveller Women's Experiences," 249.

30 Loretta J. Ross and Rickie Solinger, *Reproductive Justice: An Introduction* (Berkeley: University of California Press, 2017), 117, https://doi.org/10.1525/j.ctv1wxsth.

31 R. McConnell, S. Meaney, and K. O'Donoghue, "Influence of Cost on Contraceptive Choices Amongst University Students—Irish Medical Journal," *Irish Medical Journal* 114, no. 6 (2021): P376, http://imj.ie/influence-of-cost-on-contraceptive-choices-amongst-university-students/.

32 Government of Ireland, "Report of the Working Group on Access to Contraception," 10.

33 Luigi Barlassina, "Views and Attitudes of Oral Contraceptive Users towards the Their Availability without a Prescription in the Republic of Ireland," *Pharmacy Practice* 13, no. 2 (2015): 565–65, https://doi.org/10.18549/PharmPr act.2015.02.565; Government of Ireland, "Report of the Working Group on Access to Contraception," 15.

34 *In Her Shoes*, June 4, 2018, https://www.facebook.com/InHerIrishShoes/pho tos/a.142348133106279/168529007154858/.

35 Gordon Deegan, "Financial Barriers Remain to Effective Contraception in Ireland, Study Says," *BreakingNews.ie*, June 24, 2021, https://www.breakingn ews.ie/ireland/financial-barriers-remain-to-effective-contraception-in-ireland-study-says-1146939.html; McConnell, Meaney, and O'Donoghue, "Influence of Cost on Contraceptive Choices."

36 Government of Ireland, "Report of the Working Group on Access to Contraception," 3.

37 "Final Report on the Eighth Amendment of the Constitution—The Citizens' Assembly," accessed January 3, 2022, https://2016-2018.citizensassembly.ie/ en/The-Eighth-Amendment-of-the-Constitution/Final-Report-on-the-Eighth-Amendment-of-the-Constitution/.

38 Beth Sundstrom and Cara Delay, *Birth Control: What Everyone Needs to Know* (New York: Oxford University Press, 2020), 33–37.

39 Leigh-Ann Sweeney et al., "A Qualitative Study of Prescription Contraception Use: The Perspectives of Users, General Practitioners and Pharmacists," *PLOS ONE* 10, no. 12 (2015): e0144074, https://doi.org/10.1371/journal. pone.0144074.

40 Barbara Mintzes and Teresa Leonardo Alves, "Hormonal Contraceptives: Communication for Risk Awareness and Informed Choice, or a Public Scare?," in *Communicating about Risks and Safe Use of Medicines*, ed. P. Bahri (Adis, Singapore: Springer Singapore, 2020), 87–129, https://doi.org/ 10.1007/978-981-15-3013-5_2.

41 Laura O'Mahony et al., "Hormonal Contraceptive Use in Ireland: Trends and Co-prescribing Practices," *British Journal of Clinical Pharmacology* 80, no. 6 (2015): 1315, https://doi.org/10.1111/bcp.12755; D. Williams et al., "Effect of the British Warning on Contraceptive Use in the General Medical Service in Ireland," *Irish Medical Journal* 91, no. 6 (December 1998): 202–3.

42 Elyse Lackie and Amy Fairchild, "The Birth Control Pill, Thromboembolic Disease, Science and the Media: A Historical Review of the Relationship," *Contraception* 94, no. 4 (October 1, 2016): 295–302, https://doi.org/10.1016/ j.contraception.2016.06.009.

43 Mireille Le Guen et al., "Reasons for Rejecting Hormonal Contraception in Western Countries: A Systematic Review," *Social Science & Medicine* 284 (September 2021): 114247, https://doi.org/10.1016/j.socsci med.2021.114247.

44 Elizabeth Arveda Kissling, "What Does Not Kill You Makes You Stronger: Young Women's Online Conversations about Quitting the Pill," in *Reframing Reproduction: Conceiving Gendered Experiences*, ed. Meredith Nash (London: Palgrave Macmillan UK, 2014), 236, https://doi.org/10.1057/9781137267139_15.

45 Sweeney et al., "A Qualitative Study of Prescription Contraception Use," 6.

46 The remaining six counties on the island remained part of the United Kingdom.

47 Noel Whitty, "Law and the Regulation of Reproduction in Ireland: 1922–1992," *The University of Toronto Law Journal* 43, no. 4 (October 1, 1993): 852, https://doi.org/10.2307/825767.

48 Mary Daly, "Marriage, Fertility and Women's Lives in Twentieth-Century Ireland (c. 1900–c. 1970)," *Women's History Review* 15, no. 4 (2006): 571–85; Paul Michael Garrett, "'Unmarried Mothers' in the Republic of Ireland," *Journal of Social Work* 16, no. 6 (November 2016): 708; Maria Luddy, "Unmarried Mothers in Ireland, 1880–1973," *Women's History Review* 20, no. 1 (February 2011): 109–26.

49 Lindsay Earner-Byrne, "Moral Prescription: The Irish Medical Profession, the Roman Catholic Church and the Prohibition of Birth Control in Twentieth-Century Ireland," in *Cultures of Care in Irish Medical History, 1750–1970*, ed. Catherine Cox and Maria Luddy (New York: Palgrave Macmillan, 2010), 207–28.

50 Ireland and Committee on Evil Literature, *Report of the Committee on Evil Literature* (Dublin: Stationery Office, 1926).

51 Memo from Dept. of Posts and Telegraphs, May 10, 1926. Dept. of Justice Evil Literature Committee Files. File JUS 7/2/17, 1926, National Archives of Ireland, Dublin.

52 Houses of the Oireachtas, "Criminal Law Amendment Act, 1935—No. 6 of 1935—Houses of the Oireachtas," text, June 21, 1934, Ireland, https://www.oireachtas.ie/en/bills/bill/1934/31.

53 Sandra McAvoy, "'A Perpetual Nightmare': Women, Fertility Control, the Irish State, and The 1935 Ban on Contraceptives," in *Gender and Medicine in Ireland: 1700–1950*, ed. Margaret H. Preston and Margaret Ó hÓgartaigh (Syracuse, NY: Syracuse University Press, 2012), 189.

54 "Humanae Vitae (July 25, 1968) | Paul VI," accessed December 15, 2021, https://www.vatican.va/content/paul-vi/en/encyclicals/documents/hf_p-vi_enc_25071968_humanae-vitae.html.

55 Patrick Cooney, speech, quoted in Family Planning Association Newsletter, March 30, 1979. File BL/F/AP/1291 [1974–1979], Attic Press Archives, Boole Library, University College Cork.

56 *In Her Shoes*, April 10, 2018, https://www.facebook.com/InHerIrishShoes/photos/a.142348133106279/161106194563806/.

57 Side, "The Effects of 'Geographies of Accommodation' on Sexual and Reproductive Healthcare."

58 Health Services Executive (HSE), "Female Sterilization," *HSE.ie*, accessed November 19, 2022, https://www2.hse.ie/conditions/female-sterilisation/.

59 Conlon, O'Connor, and Ní Chatháin, "Attitudes to Fertility," 107.

60 Leslie Sherlock, "Sociopolitical Influences on Sexuality Education in Sweden and Ireland," *Sex Education* 12, no. 4 (September 2012): 383–96, https://doi.org/10.1080/14681811.2012.686882; Abbey Hyde et al., "Parents' Constructions of Communication with Their Children about Safer Sex," *Journal of Clinical Nursing* 22, no. 23–24 (December 2013): 3438–46, https://doi.org/10.1111/jocn.12367.

61 Caroline Kelleher et al., "Parental Involvement in Sexuality Education: Advancing Understanding through an Analysis of Findings from the 2010 Irish Contraception and Crisis Pregnancy Study," *Sex Education* 13, no. 4 (July 1, 2013): 463, https://doi.org/10.1080/14681811.2012.760448.

62 *In Her Shoes*, August 20, 2018, https://www.facebook.com/InHerIrishShoes/photos/a.142348133106279/236303447044080/.

63 *In Her Shoes*, September 10, 2018, https://www.facebook.com/InHerIrishShoes/photos/a.142348133106279/239381526736272.

64 *In Her Shoes*, August 29, 2018, https://www.facebook.com/InHerIrishShoes/photos/a.142348133106279/236296350378123/.

65 *In Her Shoes*, May 9, 2018, https://www.facebook.com/InHerIrishShoes/photos/a.142348133106279/167480343926391.

66 Laura Kelly, "The Contraceptive Pill in Ireland c. 1964–79: Activism, Women and Patient–Doctor Relationships," *Medical History* 64, no. 2 (April 2020): 195–218, https://doi.org/10.1017/mdh.2020.3.

67 Deirdre Foley, "'Too Many Children?' Family Planning and *Humanae Vitae* in Dublin, 1960–72," *Irish Economic and Social History* 46, no. 1 (2019): 143–44, https://doi.org/10.1177/0332489319880677.

68 Foley, "Too Many Children?," 146; Leanne McCormick, "'The Scarlet Woman in Person': The Establishment of a Family Planning Service in Northern Ireland, 1950–1974," *Social History of Medicine* 21, no. 2 (August 1, 2008): 345–60, https://doi.org/10.1093/shm/hkn028.

69 Kelly, "The Contraceptive Pill in Ireland," 210–11.

70 Laura Kelly, "Debates on Family Planning and the Contraceptive Pill in the Irish Magazine Woman's Way, 1963–1973," *Women's History Review* 30, no. 6 (2021): 971–89, https://doi.org/10.1080/09612025.2020.1833495.

71 Linda Connolly, "The Women's Movement in Ireland, 1970–1995: A Social Movements Analysis," *Irish Journal of Feminist Studies* 1, no. 1 (1996): 6, 30.

72 Connolly, "The Women's Movement in Ireland," 45.

73 Kelly, "The Contraceptive Pill in Ireland," 199; Cormac Ó Grada, *Ireland before and after the Famine: Explorations in Economic History, 1800–1925*, 2nd ed. (Manchester: Manchester University Press, 1993), 191–92.

74 Connolly, "The Women's Movement in Ireland"; Mary Minihan, "Laying the Tracks to Liberation: The Original Contraceptive Train," *The Irish Times*, October 28, 2014, https://www.irishtimes.com/news/social-affairs/laying-the-tracks-to-liberation-the-original-contraceptive-train-1.1979907.

75 Conlon, O'Connor, and Ní Chatháin, "Attitudes to Fertility," 104.

76 Delay and Sundstrom, "'In Her Shoes' and In Her Words.".

77 Katherine Side, "'A Hundred Little Violences, a Hundred Little Wounds': Personal Disclosure, Shame, and Privacy in Ireland's Abortion Access," *Éire-Ireland* 56, no. 3 (2021): 193, https://doi.org/10.1353/eir.2021.0020.

78 Sweeney et al., "A Qualitative Study of Prescription Contraception Use."

79 O'Mahony et al., "Hormonal Contraceptive Use in Ireland."

80 Begas, "New Research Shows."

81 *In Her Shoes*, April 20, 2018, https://www.facebook.com/InHerIrishShoes/photos/a.142348133106279/159928431348249/.

82 *In Her Shoes*, September 8, 2018, https://www.facebook.com/InHerIrishShoes/photos/a.142348133106279/239115680096190/.

83 *In Her Shoes*, February 5, 2018, https://www.facebook.com/InHerIrishShoes/photos/a.142348133106279/146731179334641/.

84 *In Her Shoes*, February 22, 2018, https://www.facebook.com/InHerIrishShoes/photos/a.142348133106279/150508118956947.

85 *In Her Shoes*, September 23, 2018, https://www.facebook.com/InHerIrishShoes/photos/a.142348133106279/239134280094330/.

86 O'Mahony et al., "Hormonal Contraceptive Use in Ireland."

87 Kai J. Buhling et al., "Understanding the Barriers and Myths Limiting the Use of Intrauterine Contraception in Nulliparous Women: Results of a Survey of European/Canadian Healthcare Providers," *European Journal of Obstetrics & Gynecology and Reproductive Biology* 183 (2014): 146–54, https://doi.org/10.1016/j.ejogrb.2014.10.020.

88 Sweeney et al., "A Qualitative Study of Prescription Contraception Use," 6.

89 Sweeney et al., "A Qualitative Study of Prescription Contraception Use," 8.

90 Sweeney et al., "A Qualitative Study of Prescription Contraception Use."

91 *In Her Shoes*, July 24, 2018, https://www.facebook.com/InHerIrishShoes/photos/a.142348133106279/171498833524542.

92 Sundstrom and Delay, *Birth Control*, 29, 77.

93 Marsha Kaitz, David Mankuta, and Lihi Mankuta, "Long-acting Reversible Contraception: A Route to Reproductive Justice or Injustice," *Infant Mental Health Journal* 40, no. 5 (2019): 673–89, https://doi.org/10.1002/imhj.21801.

94 Reid and Taylor, "A Feminist Exploration of Traveller Women's Experiences."

95 McBride, Morgan, and Mc Gee, "Irish Contraception and Crisis Pregnancy Study 2010," 4.

96 "Let's Talk about Sex: Here's Everything We Got up to at Our UCC #MyMorningAfter Panel," *Her.ie*, accessed January 3, 2023, https://www.her.ie/life/talk-sex-everything-ucc-mymorningafter-panel-485235.

97 Government of Ireland, "Report of the Working Group on Access to Contraception," 3–4.

98 Reid and Taylor, "A Feminist Exploration of Traveller Women's Experiences," 249.

Chapter 3

1 Houses of the Oireachtas, "Health (Regulation of Termination of Pregnancy) Act 2018—No. 31 of 2018—Houses of the Oireachtas," text, September 27, 2018, Ireland, https://www.oireachtas.ie/en/bills/bill/2018/105.

2 Fiona de Londras and Mairead Enright, *Repealing the 8th* (Bristol: Policy Press, 2018); Deirdre Niamh Duffy, "From Feminist Anarchy to Decolonization: Understanding Abortion Health Activism before and after the Repeal of the 8th Amendment," *Feminist Review* 124, no. 1 (2020): 69–85, https://doi.org/10.1177/0141778919895498; Máiréad Enright, "Four Pieces on Repeal: Notes on Art, Aesthetics and the Struggle Against Ireland's Abortion Law," *Feminist Review* 124, no. 1 (March 1, 2020): 104–23, https://doi.org/10.1177/0141778919897583; Camilla Fitzsimons, Ruth Coppinger, and Sinéad Kennedy, *Repealed: Ireland's Unfinished Fight for Reproductive Rights* (London: Pluto Press, 2021); Katie Mishler, "'It's Most Peculiar that This Particular Story Doesn't Get Told': A Reproductive-Justice Analysis of Storytelling in the Repeal Campaign in Ireland, 2012–18," *Éire-Ireland* 56, no. 3/4 (Fall/Winter 2021): 80–103.

3 Claire Bracken and Cara Delay, "Editors' Introduction: Women's Health and Reproductive Justice in Ireland," *Éire-Ireland* 56, no. 3/4 (Fall/Winter 2021): 5–20.

4 *In Her Shoes*, February 27, 2018, https://www.facebook.com/InHerIrishShoes/photos/a.142348133106279/150175165656909/.

5 Jo Murphy-Lawless, *Reading Birth and Death: A History of Obstetric Thinking* (Cork: Cork University Press, 1998).

6 Expert Government of the United Kingdom, "Offences Against the Person Act 1861," Text, 1861, https://www.legislation.gov.uk/ukpga/Vict/24-25/100/contents.

7 Cara Delay, "Kitchens and Kettles: Domestic Spaces, Ordinary Things, and Female Networks in Irish Abortion History, 1922–1949," *Journal of Women's History* 30, no. 4 (2018): 11–34; Cara Delay, "Pills, Potions, and

Purgatives: Women and Abortion Methods in Ireland, 1900–1950," *Women's History Review* 28, no. 3 (April 16, 2019): 479–99, https://doi.org/10.1080/09612025.2018.1493138; Sandra McAvoy, "Before Cadden: Abortion in Mid-Twentieth-Century Ireland," in *The Lost Decade: Ireland in the 1950s*, ed. Dermot Keogh, Finbarr O'Shea, and Carmel Quinlan (Cork: Mercier Press, 2004), 147–63; Cliona Rattigan, "'Crimes of Passion of the Worst Character': Abortion Cases and Gender in Ireland, 1925–50," in *Gender and Power in Irish History*, ed. Maryann Gialanella Valiulis (Dublin: Irish Academic Press, 2009), 115–39.

8 McAvoy, "Before Cadden."

9 Court of Criminal Appeal File CCA/36/56; Cadden Death Sentence File, Department of the Taoiseach, file S16116. Both at National Archives of Ireland, Dublin.

10 Delay, "Pills, Potions, and Purgatives."

11 Ann Rossiter, *Ireland's Hidden Diaspora: The Abortion Trail and the Making of a London-Irish Underground, 1980–2000* (London: Irish Abortion Solidarity Campaign, 2009); Medb Ruane, *The Irish Journey: Women's Stories of Abortion* (Dublin: Irish Family Planning Association, 2000).

12 Suzanna Chan, "Speaking of Silence, Speaking of Art, Abortion and Ireland," *Irish Studies Review* 27, no. 1 (February 2019): 78, https://doi.org/10.1080/09670882.2018.1560892.

13 Caelainn Hogan, *Republic of Shame: Stories from Ireland's Institutions for "Fallen Women"* (Dublin: Penguin Ireland, 2019).

14 Clara Fischer, "Abortion and Reproduction in Ireland: Shame, Nation-Building and the Affective Politics of Place," *Feminist Review* 122, no. 1 (2019): 33, https://doi.org/10.1177/0141778919850003.

15 *In Her Shoes*, August 30, 2018, https://www.facebook.com/InHerIrishShoes/photos/a.142348133106279/236303447044080/.

16 *In Her Shoes*, July 29, 2018, https://www.facebook.com/InHerIrishShoes/photos/a.142348133106279/207812553226503/.

17 Lindsey Earner-Byrne and Diane Urquhart, *The Irish Abortion Journey, 1920–2018* (New York: Palgrave Macmillan, 2019).

18 Ruane, *The Irish Journey*, 44.

19 Michaela Carroll et al., "'Our Darkest Hour': Women and Structural Violence under Ireland's 8th Amendment," *Feminist Encounters* 6, no. 1 (2022), 12.

20 Cara Delay, "Wrong for Womankind and the Nation: Anti-Abortion Discourses in 20th-Century Ireland," *Journal of Modern European History* 17, no. 3 (August 2019): 322, https://doi.org/10.1177/1611894419854660.

21 Delay, "Wrong for Womankind and the Nation," 313.

22 Delay, "Wrong for Womankind and the Nation," 322.

23 Wendy Holden, *Unlawful Carnal Knowledge: The True Story of the Irish "X" Case* (London: Harper Collins, 1994); "X Case Defined State Law on Abortion," *The*

Irish Times, February 18, 2002, https://www.irishtimes.com/news/x-case-defi ned-state-law-on-abortion-1.1050769.

24 Katherine Side, "A. B. and C. versus Ireland A New Beginning to Access Abortion in the Republic of Ireland?," *International Feminist Journal of Politics* 13, no. 3 (2011): 390–412, https://doi.org/10.1080/14616742.2011.587370.

25 Lisa Smyth, "Narratives of Irishness and the Problem of Abortion: The X Case 1992," *Feminist Review* 60, no. 1 (1998): 61–83, https://doi.org/10.1080/0141 77898339398.

26 Side, "A. B. and C. versus Ireland," 391.

27 Earner-Byrne and Urquhart, *The Irish Abortion Journey*, 111–12.

28 Kitty Holland, "How the Death of Savita Halappanavar Revolutionized Ireland," *The Irish Times*, May 28, 2018, https://www.irishtimes.com/news/social-affa irs/how-the-death-of-savita-halappanavar-revolutionised-ireland-1.3510387.

29 David Ralph, *Abortion and Ireland: How the 8th Was Overthrown* (London: Palgrave Pivot, 2020), 46, https://doi.org/10.1007/978-3-030-58692-8.

30 Sinead O'Carroll, "Savita Tragedy Continues to Attract International Attention," *TheJournal.ie*, November 15, 2012, https://www.thejournal.ie/international-media-savita-675478-Nov2012/.

31 Amelia Gentleman, "UN Calls on Ireland to Reform Abortion Laws after Landmark Ruling," *The Guardian*, June 9, 2016, https://www.theguardian.com/world/2016/jun/09/ireland-abortion-laws-violated-human-rights-says-un.

32 Government of Ireland, "About the Citizens Assembly," https://2016-2018. citizensassembly.ie/en/About-the-Citizens-Assembly/

33 Ralph, *Abortion and Ireland*, 47.

34 Mishler, "'It's Most Peculiar that This Particular Story Doesn't Get Told'," 80.

35 "Who We Are," *Together for Yes*, accessed January 3, 2023, https://www.togethe rforyes.ie/about-us/who-we-are/.

36 Gráinne Healy, *Ireland Says Yes: The inside Story of How the Vote for Marriage Equality Was Won* (Dublin: Merrion Press, 2016), 40.

37 Ralph, *Abortion and Ireland*.

38 Rachael A. Young, "'We Can't Keep Painting Over Our Problems': Murals, Social Media, and Feminist Activism in Ireland," *Éire-Ireland* 56, no. 3 (2021): 321, https://doi.org/10.1353/eir.2021.0012.

39 Enright, "Four Pieces on Repeal"; Niamh NicGhabhann, "City Walls, Bathroom Stalls and Tweeting the Taoiseach: The Aesthetics of Protest and the Campaign for Abortion Rights in the Republic of Ireland," *Continuum* 32, no. 5 (September 3, 2018): 553–68, https://doi.org/10.1080/10304312.2018.1468413; Lorna O'Hara, "Exploring 'Artivist' Innovations in Ireland's pro-Choice Campaign," *Soundings (London, England)* 76, no. 76 (2020): 50, https://doi.org/10.3898/SOUN.76.03.2020.

40 Enright, "Four Pieces on Repeal," 110.

41 NicGhabhann, "City Walls, Bathroom Stalls and Tweeting the Taoiseach," 555.

42 Young, "We Can't Keep Painting Over Our Problems."

43 *In Her Shoes*, April 20, 2018, https://www.facebook.com/InHerIrishShoes/photos/a.142348133106279/160626374611788/.

44 *In Her Shoes*, February 6, 2018, https://www.facebook.com/InHerIrishShoes/photos/a.142348133106279/146931895981236/.

45 *In Her Shoes*, March 11, 2018, https://www.facebook.com/InHerIrishShoes/photos/a.142348133106279/154281678579591/.

46 *In Her Shoes*, January 23, 2018, https://www.facebook.com/InHerIrishShoes/photos/a.142348133106279/144163986258027/.

47 *In Her Shoes*, January 23, 2018, https://www.facebook.com/InHerIrishShoes/photos/a.142348133106279/144163986258027.

48 *In Her Shoes*, April 11, 2018, https://www.facebook.com/InHerIrishShoes/photos/a.142348133106279/162142321126860/.

49 *In Her Shoes*, June 1, 2018, https://www.facebook.com/InHerIrishShoes/photos/a.142348133106279/170747610266331/.

50 Mishler, "'It's Most Peculiar that This Particular Story Doesn't Get Told'," 84; Loretta Ross and Rickie Solinger, *Reproductive Justice: An Introduction* (Oakland: University of California Press, 2017), 59.

51 Hyesun Hwang and Kee-Ok Kim, "Social Media as a Tool for Social Movements: The Effect of Social Media Use and Social Capital on Intention to Participate in Social Movements," *International Journal of Consumer Studies* 39, no. 5 (2015): 478–88, https://doi.org/10.1111/ijcs.12221.

52 Bracken and Delay, "Editors' Introduction."

53 Katherine Side, "'A Hundred Little Violences, a Hundred Little Wounds': Personal Disclosure, Shame, and Privacy in Ireland's Abortion Access," *Éire-Ireland* 56, no. 3 (2021): 198, https://doi.org/10.1353/eir.2021.0020.

54 Side, "A Hundred Little Violences," 191.

55 Paul Hosford, "Facebook Page Where Women Tell Their Abortion Stories Deliberately Sabotaged in Online Attack," *The Journal*, April 4, 2018, https://www.thejournal.ic/in-her-shoes-fb-page-3939172-Apr2018/.

56 Brian Leonard, "My Repeal(Shield) Story," *Abortion Rights Campaign*, May 19, 2020, https://www.abortionrightscampaign.ie/2020/05/19/my-repealshield-story/.

57 Rachel Lavin and Roland Adorjani, "How Ireland Beat Dark Ads," *Foreign Policy*, June 1, 2018, https://foreignpolicy.com/2018/06/01/abortion-referendum-how-ireland-resisted-bad-behaviour-online/.

58 Lavin and Adorjani, "How Ireland Beat Dark Ads."

59 Urooba Jamal, "Poland Abortion Laws: Woman's Death Spurs Calls for Change | Women's Rights News," *Al Jazeera*, December 1, 2021, https://www.aljazeera.com/news/2021/12/1/poland-abortion-laws-womans-death-spurs-calls-for-change.

60 Side, "A Hundred Little Violences," 184–85.

61 Joanne Conaghan, "Some Reflections on Law and Gender in Modern Ireland," *Feminist Legal Studies* 27, no. 3 (2019): 335, https://doi.org/10.1007/s10 691-019-09415-0.

62 Linda Connolly, *The Irish Women's Movement: From Revolution to Devolution* (New York: Palgrave, 2002); Sandra McAvoy, "From Anti-Amendment Campaigns to Demanding Reproductive Justice: The Changing Landscape of Abortion Rights Activism in Ireland, 1983–2008," in *The Unborn Child, Article 40.3.3 and Abortion in Ireland: Twenty-Five Years of Protection?*, ed. Jennifer Schweppe (Dublin: The Liffey Press, 2009), 15–45; Mary Muldowney, "Breaking the Silence on Abortion: The 1983 Referendum Campaign," *History Ireland* 21, no. 2 (2013): 42–45; Anne Speed, "The Struggle for Reproductive Rights: A Brief History in Its Political Context," in *The Abortion Papers: Ireland*, ed. Ailbhe Smyth (Dublin: Attic Press, 1992).

63 Laura Kelly, "Irishwomen United, the Contraception Action Programme and the Feminist Campaign for Free, Safe and Legal Contraception in Ireland, c.1975–81," *Irish Historical Studies* 43, no. 164 (November 2019): 273, https:// doi.org/10.1017/ihs.2019.54.

64 Sally Sheldon, "How Can a State Control Swallowing? The Home Use of Abortion Pills in Ireland," *Reproductive Health Matters* 24, no. 48 (2016): 92, https://doi.org/10.1016/j.rhm.2016.10.002.

65 Alyssa Best, "Abortion Rights along the Irish-English Border and the Liminality of Women's Experiences," *Dialectical Anthropology* 29, no. 3/4 (September 2005): 423.

66 Aideen Catherine O'Shaughnessy, "Triumph and Concession? The Moral and Emotional Construction of Ireland's Campaign for Abortion Rights," *European Journal of Women's Studies* 29, no. 2 (2022), 233–49, https://doi.org/10.1177/ 13505068211040999.

67 Anja Nyberg, "Achieving Reproductive Justice: Some Implications of Race for Abortion Activism in Northern Ireland," *Feminist Review* 124, no. 1 (March 1, 2020): 165, https://doi.org/10.1177/0141778919894912.

68 Mishler, "'It's Most Peculiar that This Particular Story Doesn't Get Told,'" 94.

69 "On Migrant Women and the 8th Amendment," *MERJ—Migrants and Ethnic-minorities for Reproductive Justice*, accessed December 14, 2021, https://merjirel and.org/index.php/2019/02/05/migrant-women-and-the-8th-amendment/.

70 Beulah Ezeugo, "Archiving Marginalized Communities," *Archiving the 8th* (blog), September 1, 2021, https://archivingthe8th.ucd.ie/collecting/margi nalised-communities/.

71 Fitzsimons, Coppinger, and Kennedy, *Repealed*, 14.

72 "What Does Reproductive Justice Look Like after the Referendum? A Migrant Perspective," *MERJ* (blog), accessed December 14, 2021, https://merjireland. org/index.php/2019/02/05/what-does-reproductive-justice-look-like-after-the-referendum-a-migrant-perspective/.

73 Cate McCurry, "Ireland's Abortion Laws 'Still Failing Women Who Struggle to Access Services," *Independent.ie*, January 3, 2022, https://www.independent.ie/breaking-news/irish-news/irelands-abortion-laws-still-failing-women-who-struggle-to-access-services-41204748.html.

74 Alison Spillane et al., "Early Abortion Care during the COVID-19 Public Health Emergency in Ireland: Implications for Law, Policy, and Service Delivery," *International Journal of Gynecology and Obstetrics* 154, no. 2 (August 2021): 379–84, https://doi.org/10.1002/ijgo.13720.

75 Spillane et al., "Early Abortion Care."

76 Spillane et al., "Early Abortion Care."

77 Beau Donnelly, "Parts of Ireland Do Not Have Equal Access to Abortion Three Years on from Vote," *The Times*, December 9, 2021, https://www.thetimes.co.uk/article/parts-of-ireland-do-not-have-equal-access-to-abortion-three-years-on-from-vote-kkt8q9lz3.

78 *Archiving the 8th* (blog), accessed January 26, 2022, https://archivingthe8th.ucd.ie/.

Chapter 4

1 Susan McKay, "Ireland's Feminists Lost the Abortion Argument in '83. This Time We Can," *The New York Times*, May 5, 2018, https://www.nytimes.com/2018/05/05/opinion/sunday/ireland-abortion-referendum.html.

2 John Spain, "'Get Your Rosaries off My Ovaries'—The Catholic Church v Ireland's New Maternity Hospital," *Irish Central*, July 9, 2021, https://www.irishcentral.com/opinion/others/catholic-church-v-irelands-new-maternity-hospital.

3 Aengus Cox, "Extended Lease Proposed for New National Maternity Hospital," *RTÉ*, October 23, 2021, https://www.rte.ie/news/ireland/2021/1023/1255536-national-maternity-hospital/.

4 Cox, "Extended Lease Proposal."

5 Caitriona Clear, *Women of the House: Women's Household Work in Ireland, 1922–1961* (Dublin: Irish Academic Press, 2000); Cara Delay, "Women, Childbirth Customs and Authority in Ireland, 1850–1930," *Lilith*, no. 21 (August 2015): 6–18.

6 Ciara Breathnach, "Handywomen and Birthing in Rural Ireland, 1851–1955," *Gender & History* 28, no. 1 (April 2016): 34–56, https://doi.org/10.1111/1468-0424.12176.

7 "Recollections of Kathleen Sheehan (1894–1985), County Cavan," in *No Shoes in Summer: Days to Remember*, ed. Mary Ryan, Seán Browne, and Kevin Gilmour (Dublin: Wolfhound Press, 1995), 89.

8 Ciara Breathnach, "Lady Dudley's District Nursing Scheme and the Congested District Boards, 1903–1923," in *Gender and Medicine in Ireland, 1700–1950*, ed. Margaret H. Preston and Margaret Ó hÓgartaigh (Syracuse, NY: Syracuse University Press, 2012), 139–153; Ciara Breathnach, "The Triumph of Proximity: The Impact of District Nursing Schemes in 1890s' Rural Ireland," *Nursing History Review* 26, no. 1 (January 2018): 68–82, https://doi.org/10.1891/1062-8061.26.68; Gerard M. Fealy, ed., *Care to Remember: Nursing and Midwifery in Ireland* (Cork: Mercier Press, 2005); Margaret Ó hÓgartaigh, "Flower Power and 'Mental Grooviness': Nurses and Midwives in Ireland in the Early Twentieth Century," in *Women in Paid Work in Ireland, 1500–1930* (Dublin: Four Courts Press, 2000), 133–47.

9 Cara Delay, "'In All Circumstances': Home Births and Collaborative Healthcare in Ireland, 1900–1950," forthcoming in *Bulletin of the History of Medicine.*

10 Sylda Langford, *Creating a Better Future Together: National Maternity Strategy 2016–2026* (Dublin: Department of Health, 2016), https://www.gov.ie/en/publication/0ac5a8-national-maternity-strategy-creating-a-better-future-together-2016-2/.

11 Andrew Hunter et al., "Woman-Centered Care during Pregnancy and Birth in Ireland: Thematic Analysis of Women's and Clinicians' Experiences," *BMC Pregnancy and Childbirth* 17, no. 1 (September 25, 2017): 322, https://doi.org/10.1186/s12884-017-1521-3.

12 Langford, *Creating a Better Future Together.*

13 Langford, *Creating a Better Future Together.*

14 Paddy Gillespie et al., "An Analysis of Antenatal Care Pathways to Mode of Birth in Ireland," *The Economic and Social Review* 50, no. 2 (June 25, 2019): 391–427.

15 Langford, *Creating a Better Future Together.*

16 Health Information and Quality Authority (HIQA), *Investigation into the safety, quality and standards of services provided by the Health Service Executive to patients, including pregnant women, at risk of clinical deterioration, including those provided in University Hospital Galway* (Dublin: Regulation of Health and Social Care Services, HIQA, 2013). https://www.hiqa.ie/sites/default/files/2017-01/Patient-Safety-Investigation-UHG.pdf

17 Langford, *Creating a Better Future Together.*

18 Health Information and Quality Authority (HIQA), *Overview Report of HIQA's Monitoring Programme against the National Standards for Safer Better Maternity Services, with a Focus on Obstetric Emergencies* (Dublin: Regulation of Health and Social Care Services, HIQA, 2020).

19 Langford, *Creating a Better Future Together*, 3.

20 Langford, *Creating a Better Future Together*, 13.

21 Denise O'Brien, Mary Casey, and Michelle M. Butler, "Women's Experiences of Exercising Informed Choices as Expressed through Their Sense of Self and Relationships with Others in Ireland: A Participatory Action Research

Study," *Midwifery* 65 (October 1, 2018): 58–66, https://doi.org/10.1016/j.midw.2018.07.006.

22 O'Brien, Casey, and Butler, "Women's Experiences of Exercising Informed Choices."

23 O'Brien, Casey, and Butler, "Women's Experiences of Exercising Informed Choices."

24 Elizabeth Rigg and Hannah Grace Dahlen, "Woman Centered Care: Has the Definition Been Morphing of Late?," *Women and Birth* 34, no. 1 (February 1, 2021): 1–3, https://doi.org/10.1016/j.wombi.2020.12.013.

25 Nicky Leap, "Woman-Centered or Women-Centered Care: Does It Matter?," *British Journal of Midwifery* 17, no. 1 (January 1, 2009): 12–16, https://doi.org/10.12968/bjom.2009.17.1.37646; Rigg and Dahlen, "Woman Centered Care."

26 HIQA, *Overview Report.*

27 Langford, *Creating a Better Future Together.*

28 Deirdre Daly et al., "The Maternal Health-Related Issues that Matter Most to Women in Ireland as They Transition to Motherhood—A Qualitative Study," *Women and Birth*, February 10, 2021, https://doi.org/10.1016/j.wombi.2021.01.013; O'Brien, Casey, and Butler, "Women's Experiences of Exercising Informed Choices"; Hunter et al., "Woman-Centered Care."

29 Hunter et al., "Woman-Centered Care."

30 Hunter et al., "Woman-Centered Care."

31 Daly et al., "The Maternal Health-Related Issues that Matter Most."

32 Daly et al., "The Maternal Health-Related Issues that Matter Most."

33 Department of Health, *Healthy Ireland: A Framework for Improved Health and Wellbeing 2013–2015* (Dublin: Department of Health). https://www.hse.ie/eng/services/publications/corporate/hienglish.pdf

34 Langford, *Creating a Better Future Together.*

35 Langford, *Creating a Better Future Together.*

36 Langford, *Creating a Better Future Together.*

37 Daly et al., "The Maternal Health-Related Issues that Matter Most."

38 Langford, *Creating a Better Future Together.*

39 Eithne Luibhéid, *Pregnant on Arrival: Making the Illegal Immigrant* (University of Minnesota Press, Minneapolis, 2013).

40 Langford, *Creating a Better Future Together.*

41 Langford, *Creating a Better Future Together.*

42 Luibhéid, *Pregnant on Arrival.*

43 Luibhéid, *Pregnant on Arrival.*

44 Luibhéid, *Pregnant on Arrival.*

45 Jill Allison, *Motherhood and Infertility in Ireland: Presence of Absence* (Cork: Cork University Press, 2013), http://muse.jhu.edu/book/27205.

46 "Fertility Treatment," *HSE.ie*, accessed January 29, 2022, https://www2.hse.ie/conditions/fertility-problems-treatments/fertility-treatment/.

47 "Fertility Treatment."

48 Evelyn Mahon and Noelle Cotter, "Assisted Reproductive Technology—IVF Treatment in Ireland: A Study of Couples with Successful Outcomes," *Human Fertility* 17, no. 3 (September 1, 2014): 165–69, https://doi.org/10.3109/14647273.2014.948498.

49 Conor O'Mahoney, *A Review of Children's Rights and Best Interests in the Context of Donor Assisted Human Reproduction and Surrogacy in Irish Law* (Dublin: Department of Children, Equality, Disability, Integration and Youth, 2021), https://www.gov.ie/en/publication/3e601-a-review-of-childrens-rig hts-and-best-interests-in-the-context-of-donorassisted-human-reproa-rev iew-of-childrens-rights-and-best-interests-in-the-context-of-donor-assis ted-human-reproduction-and-surrogacy-in-irish-law-duction-and-surrogacy-in-irish-law/.

50 O'Mahoney, *A Review of Children's Rights.*

51 Allison, *Motherhood and Infertility in Ireland.*

52 Allison, *Motherhood and Infertility in Ireland.*

53 Brendan Kennelly et al., "The COVID-19 Pandemic in Ireland: An Overview of the Health Service and Economic Policy Response," *Health Policy and Technology,* 9, no. 4 (December 1, 2020): 419–29, https://doi.org/10.1016/j.hlpt.2020.08.021.

54 Pauline Cullen and Mary P. Murphy, "Responses to the COVID-19 Crisis in Ireland: From Feminized to Feminist," *Gender, Work & Organization* 28, no. S2 (2021): 348–65, https://doi.org/10.1111/gwao.12596.

55 Cullen and Murphy, "Responses to the COVID-19 Crisis"; Rajasri G. Yaliwal et al., "Challenges of Pregnancy during the Covid19 Pandemic and Lockdown— A Cross-Sectional Study," *Pravara Medical Review* 12, no. 3 (September 2020): 23–30, https://doi.org/10.36848/PMR/2020/13100.51291.

56 Peter Beech, "The COVID-19 Pandemic Could Have Huge Knock-on Effects on Women's Health, Says the UN," *World Economic Forum,* April 2, 2020, https://www.weforum.org/agenda/2020/04/covid-19-coronavirus-pande mic-hit-women-harder-than-men/.

57 Mehreen Zaigham and Ola Andersson, "Maternal and Perinatal Outcomes with COVID-19: A Systematic Review of 108 Pregnancies," *Acta Obstetricia et Gynecologica Scandinavica* 99, no. 7 (July 2020): 823–29, https://doi.org/10.1111/aogs.13867.

58 Leah Rodriguez, "Domestic Violence Increased in the US by 8.1% During the COVID-19 Pandemic," *Global Citizen,* March 2, 2021, https://www.globalciti zen.org/en/content/domestic-violence-covid-19-increase-us-ncccj-study/.

59 Lucy S. King et al., "Pregnancy during the Pandemic: The Impact of COVID-19-Related Stress on Risk for Prenatal Depression," *Psychological Medicine,* March 30, 2021, https://doi.org/10.1017/S003329172100132X; Michael

J. McFarland et al., "Postpartum Depressive Symptoms during the Beginning of the COVID-19 Pandemic: An Examination of Population Birth Data from Central New Jersey," *Maternal & Child Health Journal*, no. 25 (January 2021): 353–59; Lauren M. Osborne, Mary C. Kimmel, and Pamela J. Surkan, "The Crisis of Perinatal Mental Health in the Age of Covid-19," *Maternal & Child Health Journal* 25, no. 3 (March 2021): 349–52, https://doi.org/10.1007/s10 995-020-03114-y.

60 Michael Ceulemans et al., "Mental Health Status of Pregnant and Breastfeeding Women during the COVID-19 Pandemic—A Multinational Cross-Sectional Study," *Acta Obstetricia et Gynecologica Scandinavica* 100, no. 7 (2021): 1219–29, https://doi.org/10.1111/aogs.14092.

61 Karen Matvienko-Sikar et al., "Differences in Levels of Stress, Social Support, Health Behaviors, and Stress-Reduction Strategies for Women Pregnant before and during the COVID-19 Pandemic, and Based on Phases of Pandemic Restrictions, in Ireland," *Women and Birth* 34, no. 5 (September 1, 2021): 447–54, https://doi.org/10.1016/j.wombi.2020.10.010.

62 N. B. Janjua et al., "COVID-19 Pandemic and Maternal Perspectives," *Irish Medical Journal* 114, no. 7 (2021): 411.

63 Sarah Cullen, Jean Doherty, and Mary Brosnan, "Women's Views on the Visiting Restrictions during COVID-19 in an Irish Maternity Hospital," *British Journal Of Midwifery* 29, no. 4 (April 2021), https://www.britishjournalofmidwifery.com/articles/women-s-views-on-the-visiting-restrictions-during-covid-19-in-an-irish-maternity-hospital/.

64 Sunita Panda et al., "Women's Views and Experiences of Maternity Care during COVID-19 in Ireland: A Qualitative Descriptive Study," *Midwifery* 103 (December 1, 2021): 103092, https://doi.org/10.1016/j.midw.2021.103092.

65 Teresa Janevic et al., "Pandemic Birthing: Childbirth Satisfaction, Perceived Health Care Bias, and Postpartum Health during the COVID-19 Pandemic," *Maternal and Child Health Journal* 25, no. 6 (June 1, 2021): 860–69, https://doi.org/10.1007/s10995-021-03158-8.

66 Ilenia Mappa, Flavia Adalgisa Distefano, and Giuseppe Rizzo, "Effects of Coronavirus 19 Pandemic on Maternal Anxiety during Pregnancy: A Prospective Observational Study," *Journal of Perinatal Medicine* 48, no. 6 (July 2020): 545–50, https://doi.org/10.1515/jpm-2020-0182.

67 Elisabeth Mahase, "COVID-19: EU States Report 60% Rise in Emergency Calls about Domestic Violence," *British Journal of Midwifery* 369 (May 11, 2020): m1872, https://doi.org/10.1136/bmj.m1872.

68 Julia Brink et al., "Intimate Partner Violence during the COVID-19 Pandemic in Western and Southern European Countries," *European Journal of Public Health* 31, no. 5 (2021), 1058–63, https://doi.org/10.1093/eurpub/ckab093.

69 King et al., "Pregnancy during the Pandemic."

70 *In Our Shoes: COVID Pregnancy*, "Updated Access Policy," November 19, 2021, https://www.facebook.com/inourshoescovidpregnancy/posts/pfbid02zRz4WS-2j8UwB6kqmrKESQY5uCdphqk5Sshf5GCnb5eBrbaT7URV9f3ayd8THg9Chl.

71 Cara Delay and Beth Sundstrom, "The Legacy of Symphysiotomy in Ireland: A Reproductive Justice Approach to Obstetric Violence," in *Reproduction, Health, and Medicine*, vol. 20 (Bingley, UK: Emerald Publishing Limited, 2019), 197–218.

72 J. Lalor et al., "Balancing Restrictions and Access to Maternity Care for Women and Birthing Partners during the COVID-19 Pandemic: The Psychosocial Impact of Suboptimal Care," *BJOG: An International Journal of Obstetrics and Gynaecology* 128, no. 11 (2021): 1720–25, https://doi.org/10.1111/1471-0528.16844.

73 Lalor et al., "Balancing Restrictions"; Anastasia Topalidou, Gill Thomson, and Soo Downe, "COVID-19 and Maternal and Infant Health: Are We Getting the Balance Right? A Rapid Scoping Review," *The Practicing Midwife* 23, no. 7 (2020): 36–25.

74 "World Patient Safety Day 2021," *World Health Organization*, September 27, 2021, https://www.who.int/news-room/events/detail/2021/09/17/default-calendar/world-patient-safety-day-2021.

75 World Health Organization, "World Patient Safety Day 2021."

76 "Ethical Framework for Respectful Maternity Care during Pregnancy and Childbirth," *FIGO: International Federation of Gynecology and Obstetrics*, September 17, 2021, https://www.figo.org/resources/figo-statements/ethical-framework-respectful-maternity-care-during-pregnancy-and-childbirth.

77 D. N. Lucas and J. H. Bamber, "Pandemics and Maternal Health: The Indirect Effects of COVID-19," *Anaesthesia* 76, no. S4 (2021): 69–75, https://doi.org/10.1111/anae.15408.

78 Michelle Sadler, Gonzalo Leiva, and Ibone Olza, "COVID-19 as a Risk Factor for Obstetric Violence," *Sexual and Reproductive Health Matters* 28, no. 1 (July 2020): 1785379, https://doi.org/10.1080/26410397.2020.1785379.

79 Lalor et al., "Balancing Restrictions."

80 Sadler, Leiva, and Olza, "COVID-19 as a Risk Factor for Obstetric Violence."

81 World Health Organization, "World Patient Safety Day 2021."

82 American College or Nurse-Midwives, "Supporting Healthy and Normal Physiologic Childbirth: A Consensus Statement by the American College of Nurse-Midwives, Midwives Alliance of North America, and the National Association of Certified Professional Midwives," *Journal of Midwifery & Women's Health* 57, no. 5 (2012): 529–32, https://doi.org/10.1111/j.1542-2011.2012.00218.x.

83 MAI Committee, *Midwives Association of Ireland: Midwives Supporting Midwives, Women, Babies, Families* (blog), August 11, 2021, https://twitter.com/MidwivesIreland/status/1425369783034392578.

84 E. Shakibazadeh et al., "Respectful Care during Childbirth in Health Facilities Globally: A Qualitative Evidence Synthesis," *International Journal of Obstetrics & Gynaecology* 125, no. 8 (2018): 932–42, https://doi.org/10.1111/1471-0528.15015.

85 *In Our Shoes*, August 21, 2021, https://www.facebook.com/inourshoescovidpregnancy/posts/pfbid02txqcH7vJz9KBQQR1VJ33LocyiwRSP6Sp7NWdarwLMr1CpzTLf6BZVHuxqwBo8aegl.

86 *In Our Shoes*, February 24, 2021, https://www.facebook.com/inourshoescovidpregnancy/posts/pfbid02kUQjn4BR8JHPiwkr8s5CJu4CAUEaiV86r-2B2GTxVjLvDeFeQhZUfbpGPRqHs63G5l

87 *In Our Shoes*, October 6, 2020, https://www.facebook.com/inourshoescovidpregnancy/posts/pfbid02g91SZWnE2C9QqsCBAV8q5xJy7eEt3G1dRbzjcoaUsfvdxPMERq51M6n8jfk1ZUqCl

88 *In Our Shoes*, October 2, 2020, https://www.facebook.com/inourshoescovidpregnancy/posts/pfbid0213okyN84ugvCD2TXEpPWFxFCxZUgvUdbiRn4noWMwHuQ6GK6REXgfxh2hwRvmqctl

89 *In Our Shoes*, February 23, 2021, https://www.facebook.com/inourshoescovidpregnancy/posts/pfbid02XLfp9gYVbB3XEiveoEsUD1LQgW254jtCggM-jgegqx6CUSULdWUTZjms1PyNdNHsul

90 *In Our Shoes*, October 2, 2020, https://www.facebook.com/inourshoescovidpregnancy/posts/pfbid02KJAMjRFyjhd5W3jKovDm5yPRktpEUTenZ1MVaWbp9T34BVzq4wwGdTEoBgRLTWC5l.

91 *In Our Shoes*, September 22, 2020, https://www.facebook.com/inourshoescovidpregnancy/photos/a.104889238030998/113613310491924

92 *In Our Shoes*, October 14, 2020, https://www.facebook.com/inourshoescovidpregnancy/posts/pfbid0KKumKtEY2J67uEpYrECf8tNcKKhoiJbSiq8YNiRYheSujTdZxDpFSGQCs7TqZaJrl

93 Patricia Larkin, Cecily M. Begley, and Declan Devane, " 'Not Enough People to Look After You': An Exploration of Women's Experiences of Childbirth in the Republic of Ireland," *Midwifery* 28, 1 (2012): 98–105.

94 *In Our Shoes*, September 26, 2020, https://www.facebook.com/inourshoescovidpregnancy/posts/pfbid02NAhzWVEHVzq2Sty4i8sJaXWha9kq2Eh7ri-AAxEyo4nhx2wo2pimoA7wbwpnPYdZDl

95 Langford, *Creating a Better Future Together*.

96 Änne Helps et al., "Impact of Bereavement Care and Pregnancy Loss Services on Families: Findings and Recommendations from Irish Inquiry Reports," *Midwifery* 91 (December 1, 2020): 102841, https://doi.org/10.1016/j.midw.2020.102841.

97 Helps et al., "Impact of Bereavement Care."

98 Helps et al., "Impact of Bereavement Care"

99 *In Our Shoes*, October 2, 2020, https://www.facebook.com/inourshoescovidpregnancy/photos/a.104956638024258/124270576092864/

100 *In Our Shoes*, December 4, 2020, https://www.facebook.com/inourshoescov idpregnancy/photos/a.104889238030998/182488020271119

101 *In Our shoes*, February 10, 2021, https://www.facebook.com/inourshoescov idpregnancy/posts/pfbid0oF4PMQJ4BvhYz8Ww1WE68S7QjQrdgEdym-WySwwzJ2mSNUKSeHrbZ8c8fGTfG77cRl

102 Nadine Edwards, Rosemary Mander, and Jo Murphy-Lawless, eds., *Untangling the Maternity Crisis* (London: Routledge, 2018).

103 Edwards, Mander, and Murphy-Lawless, *Untangling the Maternity Crisis*.

104 Delay and Sundstrom, "The Legacy of Symphysiotomy.".

105 Sadler, Leiva, and Olza, "COVID-19 as a Risk Factor for Obstetric Violence."

106 HIQA, *Overview Report*.

107 Lucas and Bamber, "Pandemics and Maternal Health."

108 Cullen and Murphy, "Responses to the COVID-19 Crisis."

109 Cullen and Murphy, "Responses to the COVID-19 Crisis."

Chapter 5

1 Upton Sinclair, *The Coal War* (New York: Open Road Integrated Media, 1976).

2 Abby Bender, "Shame and the Breastfeeding Mother in Ireland," *Éire-Ireland* 56, no. 3 (2021): 129, https://doi.org/10.1353/eir.2021.0017

3 "The Cork Survivors and Supporters Alliance (CSSA) to receive the 2021 Spirit of Mother Jones Award," *The Spirit of Mother Jones Festival*, November 23, 2021, https://motherjonescork.com/2021/11/23/the-cork-survivors-and-supporters-alliance-cssa-to-receive-the-2021-spirit-of-mother-jones-award/.

4 "Fertility," *Central Statistics Office*, https://www.cso.ie/en/releasesandpubli cations/ep/p-cp4hf/cp4hf/fty/.

5 L. McMahon et al., *Irish Maternity Indicator System National Report 2020* (Dublin: National Women and Infants Health Programme, 2021).

6 "OECD Caesarean Sections," *OECD.org*, https://data.oecd.org/healthcare/ caesarean-sections.htm.

7 "New WHO Guidance on Non-Clinical Interventions Specifically Designed to Reduce Unnecessary Caesarean Sections," *World Health Organization*, October 11, 2018), https://www.who.int/news/item/11-10-2018-new-who-guidance-on-non-clinical-interventions-specifically-designed-to-reduce-unne cessary-caesarean-sections.

8 Sylda Langford, *Creating a Better Future Together: National Maternity Strategy 2016–2026* (Dublin: Department of Health, 2016), https://www.gov.ie/ en/publication/0ac5a8-national-maternity-strategy-creating-a-better-future-together-2016-2/.

9   Marie O'Halloran, "Rise in Home Births Linked to Restrictions on Hospital Visits," *The Irish Times*, April 3, 2021, https://www.irishtimes.com/news/social-affairs/rise-in-home-births-linked-to-restrictions-on-hospital-visits-1.4527547.

10 Della Pollock, *Telling Bodies Performing Birth: Everyday Narratives of Childbirth* (New York: Columbia University Press, 1999).

11 *Rebel Women*, 1978, BL/F/AP/1295 [1978] 4 items, Attic Press archives, Boole Library, University College Cork.

12 "Irish Women United," 1979 1974, BL/F/AP/1291 [1974–1979] 3 items, Attic Press archives, Boole Library, University College Cork.

13 "Irish Women United."

14 Patricia Kennedy and Jo Murphy-Lawless, "The Maternity Care Needs of Refugee and Asylum Seeking Women in Ireland," *Feminist Review* 73, no. 1 (April 1, 2003): 39–53, https://doi.org/10.1057/palgrave.fr.9400073.

15 "Women's International Information and Communication Service," 1977, BL/F/AP/1291 [1974–1979] 3 items, Attic Press archives, Boole Library, University College Cork.

16 Zakiya Luna, *Reproductive Rights as Human Rights: Women of Color and the Fight for Reproductive Justice* (New York: NYU Press, 2020), 147.

17 O'Hare MF, Manning E, O'Herlihy C, Greene RA on behalf of MDE Ireland. Confidential Maternal Enquiry in Ireland, Data Brief No 1. Cork: MDE Ireland, December 2015. https://www.ucc.ie/en/media/research/maternaldeathenquiryireland/MDEIrelandDataBriefNo1December2015.pdf

18 Jo Murphy-Lawless, "Holding the State to Account: 'Picking Up the Threads' for Women Who Have Died in Irish Maternity Services," *Éire-Ireland* 56, no. 3 (2021): 68, https://doi.org/10.1353/eir.2021.0015.

19 P. Scranton and G. McNaull, *Death Investigation, Coroners' Inquests and the Rights of the Bereaved: A Research Report for the Irish Council for Civil Liberties* (Dublin: Irish Council for Civil Liberties, 2021).

20 Martina Hynan, "Chapter 14: Hidden in Plain Sight," in *Untangling the Maternity Crisis*, ed. Nadine Edwards, Rosemary Mander, and Jo Murphy-Lawless (London: Routledge, 2018), https://www.routledge.com/Untangling-the-Maternity-Crisis/Edwards-Mander-Murphy-Lawless/p/book/9781138244221.

21 *Migrants and Ethnic-minorities for Reproductive Justice (MERJ)*, January 12, 2018, https://www.facebook.com/MERJIreland/posts/pfbid023ZH3UjGUXs-G2aufn5iSH1HgBPEVXBqcp2ZmvbEtXEbw6GUJcSGrSmadZdsXwvEND1

22 Kitty Holland, "Families of Women Who Died in Childbirth Left in the Dark, Says Midwife," *The Irish Times*, January 30, 2019, https://www.irishtimes.com/news/social-affairs/families-of-women-who-died-in-childbirth-left-in-the-dark-says-midwife-1.3775149.

23 Department of Justice, "Minister Flanagan Announces Further Commencement of Provisions of the Coroners (Amendment) Act 2019," *Gov.ie*, January 17, 2020), https://www.gov.ie/en/press-release/a433d6-minister-flanagan-announces-further-commencement-of-provisions-of-th/.

24 Murphy-Lawless, "Holding the State to Account," 79.

25 Scranton and McNaull, "Death Investigation, Coroners' Inquests."

26 The Elephant Collective, October 7, 2021, https://www.facebook.com/permal ink.php?story_fbid=pfbid02D6yCFcJ8VPbLwHArHENKWqhqSmcnx97Uw-G1QgnEnkti2gCE9vap8MWsRv6cHc9P3l&id=1662667163990925.

27 Carolyn Tobin, Jo Murphy-Lawless, and Cheryl Tatano Beck, "Childbirth in Exile: Asylum Seeking Women's Experience of Childbirth in Ireland," *Midwifery*, 30, no. 7 (July 1, 2014): 831–38, https://doi.org/10.1016/j.midw.2013.07.012.

28 Susann Huschke, Sylvia Murphy-Tighe, and Maebh Barry, "Perinatal Mental Health in Ireland: A Scoping Review," *Midwifery* 89 (October 1, 2020): 102763, https://doi.org/10.1016/j.midw.2020.102763.

29 Gillian A. Corbett et al., "Childbirth in Ireland's Capital City over Sixty Years," *Irish Journal of Medical Science (1971-)* 189, no. 3 (August 1, 2020): 1135–41, https://doi.org/10.1007/s11845-020-02192-9.

30 Corbett et al., "Childbirh in Ireland's Capital City."

31 Jane X, "My Activism and My Experience in a Maternity Hospital in Ireland," *Migrants and Ethnic-minorities for Reproductive Justice* (blog), n.d., https://merj ireland.org/index.php/2019/04/09/my-activism-my-experience-in-a-matern ity-hospital-in-ireland/.

32 Cara Delay and Beth Sundstrom, "The Legacy of Symphysiotomy in Ireland: A Reproductive Justice Approach to Obstetric Violence," in *Reproduction, Health, and Medicine*, vol. 20 (Bingley, UK: Emerald Publishing Limited, 2019), 197–218, https://doi.org/10.1108/S1057-629020190000020017.

33 Nadine Edwards, "Chapter 7: The Trauma Women Experience as the Result of Our Current Maternity Services," in *Untangling the Maternity Crisis*, ed. Nadine Edwards, Rosemary Mander, and Jo Murphy-Lawless (London: Routledge, 2018), https://www.routledge.com/Untangling-the-Maternity-Crisis/Edwa rds-Mander-Murphy-Lawless/p/book/9781138244221.

34 Mavis Kirkham, "Chapter 9: Fundamental Contradictions," in *Untangling the Maternity Crisis*, ed. Nadine Edwards, Rosemary Mander, and Jo Murphy-Lawless (London: Routledge, 2018), https://www.routledge.com/Untangl ing-the-Maternity-Crisis/Edwards-Mander-Murphy-Lawless/p/book/978113 8244221.

35 Rosemary Mander, "Chapter 4: The BPG Survey," in *Untangling the Maternity Crisis*, ed. Nadine Edwards, Rosemary Mander, and Jo Murphy-Lawless (London: Routledge, 2018), https://www.routledge.com/Untangling-the-Maternity-Crisis/Edwards-Mander-Murphy-Lawless/p/book/978113 8244221.

36 Orla Donohoe, "Chapter 3: The BPG Survey," in *Untangling the Maternity Crisis*, ed. Nadine Edwards, Rosemary Mander, and Jo Murphy-Lawless (London: Routledge, 2018), https://www.routledge.com/Untangling-the-Maternity-Crisis/Edwards-Mander-Murphy-Lawless/p/book/978113 8244221.

37 Nadine Edwards, Rosemary Mander, and Jo Murphy-Lawless, eds., *Untangling the Maternity Crisis* (London: Routledge, 2018), https://www.routledge.com/Untangling-the-Maternity-Crisis/Edwards-Mander-Murphy-Lawless/p/book/9781138244221.

38 Patricia Larkin, Cecily M. Begley, and Declan Devane, "'Not Enough People to Look after You': An Exploration of Women's Experiences of Childbirth in the Republic of Ireland," *Midwifery* 28, no. 1 (February 1, 2012): 98–105, https://doi.org/10.1016/j.midw.2010.11.007.

39 United Nations, "Universal Declaration of Human Rights," *UN.org*, accessed January 29, 2022, https://www.un.org/en/about-us/universal-declaration-of-human-rights.

40 Edwards, Mander, and Murphy-Lawless, *Untangling the Maternity Crisis*; Larkin, Begley, and Devane, "'Not Enough People to Look after You.'"

41 Anna Dencker et al., "Childbirth Experience Questionnaire (CEQ): Development and Evaluation of a Multidimensional Instrument," *BMC Pregnancy and Childbirth* 10, no. 1 (December 10, 2010): 81, https://doi.org/10.1186/1471-2393-10-81.

42 Corbett et al., "Childbirth in Ireland's Capital City over Sixty Years."

43 Corbett et al., "Childbirth in Ireland's Capital City over Sixty Years."

44 National Institute for Health Care and Excellence (NICE), *NICE Quality Standard for Caesarean Section* (Manchester: NICE, 2013), https://www.nice.org.uk/guidance/qs32.

45 Jennifer E. Lutomski et al., "Private Health Care Coverage and Increased Risk of Obstetric Intervention," *BMC Pregnancy and Childbirth* 14, no. 1 (January 13, 2014): 13, https://doi.org/10.1186/1471-2393-14-13.

46 Patrick S. Moran et al., "Predictors of Choice of Public and Private Maternity Care among Nulliparous Women in Ireland, and Implications for Maternity Care and Birth Experience," *Health Policy* 124, no. 5 (May 1, 2020): 556–62, https://doi.org/10.1016/j.healthpol.2020.02.008.

47 Moran et al., "Predictors of Choice."

48 Katie Cook and Colleen Loomis, "The Impact of Choice and Control on Women's Childbirth Experiences," *The Journal of Perinatal Education* 21, no. 3 (January 1, 2012): 158–68, https://doi.org/10.1891/1058-1243.21.3.158; Dencker et al., "Childbirth Experience Questionnaire (CEQ)."

49 Huschke, Murphy-Tighe, and Barry, "Perinatal Mental Health in Ireland"; Larkin, Begley, and Devane, "'Not Enough People to Look after You.'"

50 Moran et al., "Predictors of Choice."

51 Ingela Lundgren et al., "Cultural Perspectives on Vaginal Birth after Previous Caesarean Section in Countries with High and Low Rates—A Hermeneutic Study," *Women and Birth* 33, no. 4 (July 1, 2020): e339–47, https://doi.org/10.1016/j.wombi.2019.07.300.

52 Helen M. Haines et al., "The Influence of Women's Fear, Attitudes and Beliefs of Childbirth on Mode and Experience of Birth," *BMC Pregnancy and Childbirth* 12, no. 1 (June 24, 2012): 55, https://doi.org/10.1186/1471-2393-12-55.

53 Mary Koehn, "Contemporary Women's Perceptions of Childbirth Education," *The Journal of Perinatal Education* 17, no. 1 (January 1, 2008): 11–18, https://doi.org/10.1624/105812408X267916; Larkin, Begley, and Devane, "'Not Enough People to Look after You.'"

54 Cook and Loomis, "The Impact of Choice and Control"; Dencker et al., "Childbirth Experience Questionnaire (CEQ)"; Koehn, "Contemporary Women's Perceptions of Childbirth Education."

55 Patricia Larkin, Cecily M. Begley, and Declan Devane, "Women's Preferences for Childbirth Experiences in the Republic of Ireland; a Mixed Methods Study," *BMC Pregnancy and Childbirth* 17, no. 1 (January 10, 2017): 19, https://doi.org/10.1186/s12884-016-1196-1.

56 Larkin, Begley, and Devane, "Women's Preferences for Childbirth Experiences."

57 Huschke, Murphy-Tighe, and Barry, "Perinatal Mental Health in Ireland."

58 M. F. O'Hare et al., *Confidential Maternal Death Enquiry in Ireland, Report for 2016–2018* (Cork: MDE Ireland, 2020).

59 O'Hare et al., *Confidential Maternal Death Enquiry.*

60 Neil Michael, "Perinatal Mortality within African Community in Ireland Needs 'Urgent' Investigation," Irish Examiner, May 8, 2021, https://www.irishexaminer.com/news/arid-40283846.html.

61 Michael, "Perinatal Mortality."

62 Michael, "Perinatal Mortality."

63 X, "My Activism and My Experience."

64 Kennedy and Murphy-Lawless, "The Maternity Care Needs."

65 Tobin, Murphy-Lawless, and Beck, "Childbirth in Exile."

66 Tobin, Murphy-Lawless, and Beck, "Childbirth in Exile."

67 Safa Abdalla et al., *All Ireland Traveller Health Study* (Dublin: University College, Dublin, 2010).

68 Bernadette Reid and Julie Taylor, "A Feminist Exploration of Traveller Women's Experiences of Maternity Care in the Republic of Ireland," *Midwifery* 23, no. 3 (September 1, 2007): 248–59, https://doi.org/10.1016/j.midw.2006.03.011.

69 "Fertility."

70 Abdalla et al., "All Ireland Traveller Health Study."

71 Abdalla et al., "All Ireland Traveller Health Study."

72 Fiona McGaughey, "Irish Travellers and Teenage Pregnancy: A Feminist, Cultural, Relativist Analysis," in *Re/Assembling the Pregnant and Parenting*

Teenager: Narratives from the Field(s), ed. Annelies Kamp and Majella McSharry (Oxford: Peter Lang, 2018), 173–94.

73 Reid and Taylor, "A Feminist Exploration of Traveller Women's Experiences."

74 Reid and Taylor, "A Feminist Exploration of Traveller Women's Experiences."

75 Reid and Taylor, "A Feminist Exploration of Traveller Women's Experiences," 256.

76 Reid and Taylor, "A Feminist Exploration of Traveller Women's Experiences."

77 Olivia Kelly, "Ireland's Level of Breastfeeding Is 'Pathetically Low,' Sabina Higgins Says: Opening of Breastival Hears Call for North and South to Invest in Breastfeeding Awareness," *The Irish Times*, August 2, 2021, https://www.irishti mes.com/news/health/ireland-s-level-of-breastfeeding-is-pathetically-low-sab ina-higgins-says-1.4636556.

78 Kelly, "Ireland's Level of Breastfeeding."

79 Bender, "Shame and the Breastfeeding Mother."

80 Linda Blum, *At the Breast: Ideologies of Breastfeeding and Motherhood in the Contemporary United States* (Boston: Beacon Press, 2000).

81 Bender, "Shame and the Breastfeeding Mother."

82 Lauren Gurrieri, Josephine Previte, and Jan Brace-Govan, "Women's Bodies as Sites of Control: Inadvertent Stigma and Exclusion in Social Marketing," *Journal of Macromarketing* 33, no. 2 (June 1, 2013): 128–43, https://doi.org/10.1177/ 0276146712469971.

83 Reid and Taylor, "A Feminist Exploration of Traveller Women's Experiences."

84 Reid and Taylor, "A Feminist Exploration of Traveller Women's Experiences."

85 Kennedy and Murphy-Lawless, "The Maternity Care Needs."

86 Bender, "Shame and the Breastfeeding Mother," 107–8.

87 Department of Children, Equality, Disability, Integration and Youth, *Final Report of the Commission of Investigation into Mother and Baby Homes* (Dublin: Government of Ireland, 2021), https://www.gov.ie/en/publication/ d4b3d-final-report-of-the-commission-of-investigation-into-mother-and-baby-homes/.

88 Cork Survivors and Supporters Alliance, May 26, 2021. https://twitter.com/ Lost900Bessboro/status/1397507384306716674

89 "Bessborough: Plan to Build at Mother and Baby Home Site Refused," *BBC News*, May 26, 2021, https://www.bbc.com/news/world-europe-57255760.

90 Corah Gernon, "Ireland's Birth Stories," *Irelandbirthstories*.ie, n.d., https:// www.irelandsbirthstories.ie/about

91 "Making Childbirth a Positive Experience: New WHO Guideline on Intrapartum Care," *World Health Organization*, February 15, 2018, https:// www.who.int/news/item/15-02-2018-making-childbirth-a-positive-exp erience.

92 Women's Health Taskforce. Women's Health Action Plan 2022–2023, Department of Health, March 2022, https://www.gov.ie/en/publication/ 232af-womens-health-action-plan-2022-2023/

Chapter 6

1 A symphysiotomy occurs when, in order to facilitate an obstructed birth, physicians cut the tissue around the joint of the symphysis pubis, severing the cartilage and unhinging the pelvis. Pubiotomy involves the cutting of the pubic bone itself. Marie O'Connor, *Bodily Harm: Symphysiotomy and Pubiotomy in Ireland, 1944–92* (Cathair na Mart: Evertype, 2010), 8. In twentieth-century Ireland, symphysiotomies were far more common than pubiotomies; in fact, evidence suggests that only a handful of pubiotomies were performed. This chapter therefore focuses primarily on symphysiotomies.

2 O'Connor, *Bodily Harm.*

3 Kellie Morgan and Nick Thompson, "'He Was Saying Me in Half': Irelands Gruesome Era of Symphysiotomy," *CNN.com*, January 30, 2015, https://edition.cnn.com/2015/01/30/europe/ireland-symphysiotomy/.

4 Caelainn Hogan, *Republic of Shame: Stories from Ireland's Institutions for "Fallen Women"* (Dublin: Penguin Ireland, 2019); Fiona McCann, *The Carceral Network in Ireland History, Agency and Resistance* (Cham: Springer International Publishing, 2020), https://doi.org/10.1007/978-3-030-42184-7; Katherine O'Donnell, Maeve O'Rourke, and Jennifer O'Mahoney, *Institutional Abuse in Ireland: Lessons from Magdalene Survivors and Legal Professionals* (Bristol: Bristol University Press, 2021), https://researchrepository.ucd.ie/handle/10197/11892; Nathalie Sebbane, *Memorializing the Magdalene Laundries: From Story to History* (Oxford: Peter Lang Ltd., International Academic Publishers, 2021).

5 Clara Fischer, "Gender, Nation, and the Politics of Shame: Magdalen Laundries and the Institutionalization of Feminine Transgression in Modern Ireland," *Signs* 41, no. 4 (2016): 821; Elaine Farrell, "'Poor Prison Flowers': Convict Mothers and Their Children in Ireland, 1853–1900," *Social History* 41, no. 2 (April 2, 2016): 171–91, https://doi.org/10.1080/03071022.2016.1144312; Conor Reidy, "Poverty, Alcohol, and the Women of the State Inebriate Reformatory in Ireland, 1900–1918," in *Women, Reform, and Resistance in Ireland, 1850–1950*, ed. Christina Brophy and Cara Delay (New York: Palgrave Macmillan, 2015), 119–38.

6 Hogan, *Republic of Shame.*

7 K. N. Klein, "Popular Media and Health: Images and Effects," in *The Routledge Handbook of Health Communication*, ed. T. L. Thompson, R. Parrott, and J. F. Nussbaum (New York: Routledge, 2011), 252–67.

8 Emily Martin, *The Woman in the Body: A Cultural Analysis of Reproduction* (Boston: Beacon Press, 2001).

9 Martin, *The Woman in the Body*, 22.

10 Jo Murphy-Lawless, "Holding the State to Account: 'Picking Up the Threads' for Women Who Have Died in Irish Maternity Services," *Éire-Ireland* 56, no. 3/4 (Fall/Winter 2021): 51–79; Claire Murray and Mary Donnelly, *Ethical and*

Legal Debates in Irish Healthcare: Confronting Complexities (Baltimore: Project Muse, 2017).

11 Sara Burke, *Irish Apartheid: Healthcare Inequality in Ireland* (Dublin: New Island, 2009), 14–15.

12 Don O'Leary, *Biomedical Controversies in Catholic Ireland* (Cork: Eryn Press, 2020), 215.

13 Lindsay Earner-Byrne, "Managing Motherhood: Negotiating a Maternity Service for Catholic Mothers in Dublin, 1930–1954," *Social History of Medicine* 19, no. 2 (2006): 272.

14 Sheila O'Connor, *Without Consent* (Dublin: Poolbeg, 2010), 3.

15 "The Prevention and Elimination of Disrespect and Abuse During Facility-Based Childbirth," *World Health Organization*, 2014, http://apps.who.int/iris/bitstream/10665/134588/1/WHO_RHR_14.23_eng.pdf?ua=1&ua=1.

16 Michelle Sadler et al., "Moving beyond Disrespect and Abuse: Addressing the Structural Dimensions of Obstetric Violence," *Reproductive Health Matters* 24, no. 47 (2016): 47–55, https://doi.org/10.1016/j.rhm.2016.04.002.

17 Carlos Herrera Vacaflor, "Obstetric Violence: A New Framework for Identifying Challenges to Maternal Healthcare in Argentina," *Reproductive Health Matters* 24, no. 47 (2016): 65–73, https://doi.org/10.1016/j.rhm.2016.05.001.

18 Farah Diaz-Tello, "Invisible Wounds: Obstetric Violence in the United States," *Reproductive Health Matters* 24, no. 47 (2016): 56–64, https://doi.org/10.1016/j.rhm.2016.04.004.

19 Sadler et al., "Moving beyond Disrespect and Abuse"; Vacaflor, "Obstetric Violence."

20 Vacaflor, "Obstetric Violence."

21 Joanna N. Erdman, "Bioethics, Human Rights, and Childbirth," Health and Human Rights Journal 17, no. 1 (2015): 43–51.

22 Meghan A. Bohren et al., "The Mistreatment of Women during Childbirth in Health Facilities Globally: A Mixed-Methods Systematic Review," *PLOS Medicine* 12, no. 6 (June 2015): 1–32, https://doi.org/10.1371/journal.pmed.1001847.

23 Simone Grilo Diniz et al., "Abuse and Disrespect in Childbirth Care as a Public Health Issue in Brazil: Origins, Definitions, Impacts on Maternal Health, and Proposals for Its Prevention," *Journal of Human Growth and Development* 25, no. 3 (October 25, 2015): 377, https://doi.org/10.7322/jhgd.106080.

24 Leah Culhane, "Reproductive Justice and the Irish Context: Towards an Egalitarian Framing of Abortion," in *The Abortion Papers Ireland: Volume 2* (Dublin: Attic Press, 2015), 67–79.

25 Hanna Laako, "Understanding Contested Women's Rights in Development: The Latin American Campaign for the Humanization of Birth and the Challenge of Midwifery in Mexico," *Third World Quarterly* 38, no. 2 (February 29, 2016): 1–18, https://doi.org/10.1080/01436597.2016.1145046.

26 Bohren et al., "The Mistreatment of Women during Childbirth"; Sadler et al., "Moving beyond Disrespect and Abuse"; Diniz et al., "Abuse and Disrespect in Childbirth Care."

27 Ann Rossiter, *Ireland's Hidden Diaspora: The Abortion Trail and the Making of a London-Irish Underground, 1980–2000* (London: Irish Abortion Solidarity Campaign, 2009).

28 Cara Delay and Beth Sundstrom, "The Legacy of Symphysiotomy in Ireland: A Reproductive Justice Approach to Obstetric Violence," in *Reproduction, Health, and Medicine*, vol. 20 (Bingley, UK: Emerald Publishing Limited, 2019), 197–218, https://doi.org/10.1108/S1057-629020190000020017.

29 James M. Smith, *Ireland's Magdalen Laundries and the Nation's Architecture of Containment* (South Bend, IN: University of Notre Dame Press, 2007).

30 Eilish O'Regan, "Neary Case: Top Doctors Are Guilty of Misconduct," *Independent.ie*, February 7, 2011, https://www.independent.ie/lifestyle/hea lth/neary-case-top-doctors-are-guilty-of-misconduct-26274473.html.

31 Maureen Harding Clark, *The Lourdes Hospital Inquiry* (Dublin: The Stationery Office, 2006), https://assets.gov.ie/11422/febc70aebb7840bb8bb65a4f6edbe fcc.pdf.

32 Joan McCarthy, Sharon Murphy, and Mark Loughrey, "Gender and Power: The Irish Hysterectomy Scandal," *Nursing Ethics* 15, no. 5 (2008): 644, https://doi. org/10.1177/0969733008092873.

33 Clark, *The Lourdes Hospital Inquiry*, 11–13.

34 Kathleen Ward, *A Violation Against Women* (Dublin: Liberties Press, 2015), 34.

35 O'Connor, *Without Consent*, 56.

36 O'Connor, *Without Consent*, 104–8.

37 Clark, *The Lourdes Hospital Inquiry*, 29.

38 Ciara Breathnach, "Handywomen and Birthing in Rural Ireland, 1851–1955," *Gender & History* 28, no. 1 (April 2016): 34–56, https://doi.org/10.1111/ 1468-0424.12176.

39 Central Midwives Board minute book, Dec 17, 1927. Microfilm reel #P220/ 207. *An Bord Altranais* Archives, University College Dublin.

40 Central Midwives Board minute book, February 13, 1919. Microfilm reel #P220/207. *An Bord Altranais* Archives, University College Dublin.

41 Rosemary Mander and Jo Murphy-Lawless, *The Politics of Maternity* (London: Taylor & Francis Group, 2013), http://ebookcentral.proquest.com/ lib/cofc/detail.action?docID=1170353.

42 Clark, *The Lourdes Hospital Inquiry*, 21.

43 McCarthy, Murphy, and Loughrey, "Gender and Power," 645.

44 S. Ong et al., "Prevalence of Hysterectomy in Ireland," *International Journal of Gynecology and Obstetrics* 69, no. 3 (2000): 243–47, https://doi.org/10.1016/ S0020-7292(00)00195-8.

45 Mothers & Babies iMag, "Symphysiotomy," *YouTube*, February 25, 2014, https://www.youtube.com/watch?v=FC6C2_9b-JY.

46 S. M. Menticoglou, "Is There a Role for Symphysiotomy in Developed Countries?," *Journal of Obstetrics & Gynaecology* 29, no. 4 (May 2009): 272–77, https://doi.org/10.1080/01443610902883338.

47 Oonagh Walsh, *Report on Symphysiotomy in Ireland 1944–1984* (Dublin: Department of Health, 2014), 38–39.

48 John F. O'Sullivan, "Caesarean Birth," *Ulster Medical Journal* 59, no. 1 (April 1990): 1–10.

49 Robert Jardine, "Discussion of Caesarean Section versus Other Methods of Delivery in Contracted Pelvis," *British Medical Journal*, September 19, 1908, 800.

50 US National Institutes of Health, "Caesarean Section - A Brief History: Part 3," Exhibitions, accessed December 15, 2016, https://www.nlm.nih.gov/exhibit ion/caesarean/part3.html.

51 Alexander W. Spain, "Symphysiotomy and Pubiotomy," *BJOG: An International Journal of Obstetrics and Gynaecology* 56, no. 4 (August 1, 1949): 576–85, https://doi.org/10.1111/j.1471-0528.1949.tb07126.x.

52 Walsh, "Report on Symphysiotomy in Ireland," 17.

53 Survivors of Symphysiotomy, "Survivors of Symphysiotomy Submission to the United Nations Committee Against Torture," September 21, 2015, https://upr doc.ohchr.org.

54 The Rotunda did perform symphysiotomies, although rarely, in the late nineteenth century. "Royal Academy of Medicine in Ireland," British Medical Journal, February 9, 1895, 306. Jacqueline Morrissey, "The Murder of Infants? Symphysiotomy in Ireland, 1944–66," *History Ireland* 20, no. 5 (2012): 44–47.

55 Éamon De Valera, architect of the 1937 constitution and staunch advocate of Catholicism, was both Taoiseach (Prime Minister) and President of Ireland for most of the years from 1932 to 1959.

56 Survivors of Symphysiotomy, "Survivors of Symphysiotomy."

57 Marge Berer, "Termination of Pregnancy as Emergency Obstetric Care: The Interpretation of Catholic Health Policy and the Consequences for Pregnant Women: An Analysis of the Death of Savita Halappanavar in Ireland and Similar Cases," Reproductive Health Matters 21, no. 41 (2013): 9–17.

58 O'Connor, *Bodily Harm*, 12.

59 Diaz-Tello, "Invisible Wounds."

60 Ibone Olza Fernández, "PTSD and Obstetric Violence," *Midwifery Today* (Spring 2013): 48–49, https://afar.info/biblio/private/2699.pdf.

61 O'Connor, *Bodily Harm*, 9.

62 Survivors of Symphysiotomy, "Survivors of Symphysiotomy."

63 Survivors of Symphysiotomy, "Survivors of Symphysiotomy."

64 Survivors of Symphysiotomy, "Survivors of Symphysiotomy."

65 Survivors of Symphysiotomy, "Survivors of Symphysiotomy."

66 Sara Cohen Shabot, "Making Loud Bodies 'Feminine': A Feminist-Phenomenological Analysis of Obstetric Violence," *Human Studies* 39, no. 2 (May 2016): 231, https://doi.org/10.1007/s10746-015-9369-x.

67 McCarthy, Murphy, and Loughrey, "Gender and Power," 645.

68 Jo Murphy-Lawless, "The Silencing of Women in Childbirth or Let's Hear It from Bartholomew and the Boys," *Women's Studies International Forum* 11, no. 4 (1988): 293–98; Jo Murphy-Lawless, *Reading Birth and Death: A History of Obstetric Thinking* (Cork: Cork University Press, n.d.).

69 Joanne Conaghan, "Some Reflections on Law and Gender in Modern Ireland," *Feminist Legal Studies* 27, no. 3 (2019): 339, https://doi.org/10.1007/s10 691-019-09415-0.

70 Clark, *The Lourdes Hospital Inquiry*, 188–89.

71 McCarthy, Murphy, and Loughrey, "Gender and Power," 646.

72 "Patients of Disgraced Neary to Be Paid ?45m in Compensation," *Independent. ie*, April 19, 2007, https://www.independent.ie/lifestyle/health/patients-of-disgraced-neary-to-be-paid-45m-in-compensation-26266335.html.

73 O'Connor, *Bodily Harm* 12.

74 Máiréad Enright, "'No. I Won't Go Back: National Time, Trauma and Legacies of Symphysiotomy in Ireland 1,'" in *Law and Time*, ed. Sian Beynon-Jones and Emily Grabham (London: Routledge, 2019), 50, https://doi.org/10.4324/9781315167695-3.

75 Survivors of Symphysiotomy, "Survivors of Symphysiotomy."

76 Breda O'Brien, "Why Did So Many Women Say They Had Symphysiotomies?," *The Irish Times*, December 15, 2016, http://www.irishtimes.com/opinion/breda-o-brien-why-did-so-many-women-say-they-had-symphysiotomies-1.2882141; "Publication of the Report of the Surgical Symphysiotomy Ex-Gratia Payment Scheme," *MerrionStreet.ie*, November 22, 2016, http://merrio nstreet.ie/en/News-Room/Releases/Publication_of_the_Report_of_the_Su rgical_Symphysiotomy_Ex-gratia_Payment_Scheme.html.

77 "Symphysiotomy in Ireland: Ireland Payment Scheme," accessed January 18, 2022, https://symphysiotomyireland.com/campaigning-for-access-to-the-law.

78 Enright, "'No. I Won't Go Back," 52.

79 Caelainn Hogan, "Mother and Baby Homes Report Contradicts Survivors' Lived Experiences," *The Irish Times*, January 14, 2021, https://www.irishtimes.com/opinion/mother-and-baby-homes-report-contradicts-survivors-lived-experiences-1.4457411.

80 Katherine O'Donnell, Maeve O'Rourke, and James M. Smith, "Editors' Introduction: Toward Transitional Justice in Ireland? Addressing Legacies of Harm," *Éire-Ireland* 55, no. 1/2 (2020): 10, https://doi.org/10.1353/eir.2020.0000.

81 Bill Rolston and Fionnuala Ní Aoláin, "Colonialism, Redress and Transitional Justice: Ireland and Beyond," *State Crime* 7, no. 2 (2018): 333, https://doi.org/10.13169/statecrime.7.2.0329.

82 International Center for Transitional Justice, "Canada," *ICTJ.org*, accessed February 28, 2011, https://www.ictj.org/our-work/regions-and-countries/canada.

83 Colin Luoma, "Closing the Cultural Rights Gap in Transitional Justice: Developments from Canada's National Inquiry into Missing and Murdered Indigenous Women and Girls," *Netherlands Quarterly of Human Rights* 39, no. 1 (2021): 31, citing Alexandra Xanthaki, "Indigenous Cultural Rights in International Law," *European Journal of Law Reform* 2, no. 3 (2000): 343.

84 Fionnuala Ní Aoláin, "The Inner and Outer Limits of Gendered Transitional Justice," *Éire-Ireland* 55, no. 1 (2020): 279, https://doi.org/10.1353/eir.2020.0012.

85 Rolston and Ní Aoláin, "Colonialism, Redress and Transitional Justice."

86 Lauren Dempster, *Transitional Justice and the "Disappeared" of Northern Ireland: Silence, Memory, and the Construction of the Past* (London: Routledge, 2019).

87 Ní Aoláin, "The Inner and Outer Limits," 282, 287.

88 Smith, *Ireland's Magdalen Laundries.*

89 Shabot, "Making Loud Bodies 'Feminine,'" 231.

90 National Women's Council of Ireland (NWCI), "Return the Records to Survivors of Symphysiotomy," *NWCI.org*, March 23, 2016, http://www.nwci.ie/index.php/learn/article/return_the_records_to_survivors_of_symphysiotomy.

Conclusion

1 Jacky Jones, "Ireland's Maternity Services: An Ongoing Horror Story," *The Irish Times*, December 12, 2016, http://www.irishtimes.com/life-and-style/health-family/ireland-s-maternity-services-an-ongoing-horror-story-1.2895135.

2 Louise Kenny, "Women-Centered Maternity Care," *The Irish Times*, December 15, 2016, http://www.irishtimes.com/opinion/letters/women-centred-maternity-care-1.2906282.

3 Sinéad O'Rourke, "Why Does #wearedelivering Hurt?," *AIMS Ireland: Association for Improvement in the Maternity Services—Ireland* (blog), December 16, 2016, http://aimsireland.ie/why-does-wearedelivering-hurt

4 Leslie Sherlock, "Towards a Reproductive Justice Model in Ireland," in *The Abortion Papers Ireland: Volume 2,* ed. Aideen Quilty, Catherine Conlon, and Sinéad Kennedy (Dublin: Attic Press, 2015), 89.

5 Haraway, Donna Jeanne. 2004. The Haraway Reader. New York, NY: Routledge.

6 Jennifer Vardeman-Winter and Amanda Sebesta, "The Problem of Intersectionality as an Approach to Digital Activism: The Women's March on Washington's Attempt to Unite All Women," *Journal of Public Relations Research* 32 (January 24, 2020): 1–23, https://doi.org/10.1080/10627 26X.2020.1716769.

7 www.transcribehealthcare.org.

8 www.womenonweb.org.

9 R. J. Gomperts et al., "Using Telemedicine for Termination of Pregnancy with Mifepristone and Misoprostol in Settings Where There Is No Access to Safe Services," *BJOG: An International Journal of Obstetrics and Gynaecology* 115, no. 9 (2008): 1171–78, https://doi.org/10.1111/j.1471-0528.2008.01787.x.

10 Jo Greene et al., "Seeking Online Telemedicine Abortion Outside the Jurisdiction from Ireland following Implementation of Telemedicine Provision Locally," *BMJ Sexual & Reproductive Health* 48 (2022): 256–66, https://doi. org/10.1136/bmjsrh-2021-201205.

11 Greene et al., "Seeking Online Telemedicine Abortion."

12 https://aidaccess.org/.

13 Abigail R. A. Aiken, Jennifer E. Starling, and Rebecca Gomperts, "Factors Associated with Use of an Online Telemedicine Service to Access Self-Managed Medical Abortion in the US," *JAMA Network Open* 4, no. 5 (May 21, 2021): e2111852, https://doi.org/10.1001/jamanetworkopen.2021.11852.

14 "Irish Doctor Says 'Women Will Die' if Roe V. Wade Overturned in US," *CBS News*, May 24, 2022, https://www.cbsnews.com/news/abortion-law-us-supr eme-court-ireland-mothers-doctor-on-life-illegal-abortion/.

15 Ivana Bacik, "As US Abortion Rights Take a Shocking Step Backwards, We Must Move Forward," *Irish Examiner*, June 25, 2022.

16 Ailbhe Smyth, "How One of Ireland's Leading Abortion Rights Activists Sees the Future of Roe," *TIME Magazine*, May 6, 2022.

17 Maeve Higgins, "What Irish Women Know," *The New York Times*, May 24, 2018.

18 https://www.womenonwaves.org.

19 "Crowdfunder: Reclaim Your Rights! A New Post-Roe Strategy," *Women on Waves*, accessed November 23, 2022, https://www.womenonwaves.org/en/ page/7730/crowdfunder-reclaim-your-rights-a-new-post-roe-strategy.

RESOURCES AND FURTHER INFORMATION

Abortion Rights Campaign

https://www.abortionrightscampaign.ie/

The Abortion Rights Campaign is a grassroots organization that works to secure free, safe, and legal abortion care across Ireland. It was one of the three groups that comprised Together for Yes and successfully campaigned to overturn the Eighth Amendment.

Aid Access

https://aidaccess.org/

Aid Access is a nonprofit organization begun by Dr. Rebecca Gomperts; its goal is to help women who have difficulty accessing abortion locally by providing information about medical abortion (abortion pills).

AIMS Ireland (Association for Improvements in Maternity Services)

http://aimsireland.ie

AIMS Ireland, founded in 2007, is an organization comprised of volunteers, mostly women who have experience with the country's maternity system. It seeks to provide information about best birth practices based on reliable research in order to improve the Irish maternity system.

AkiDwA

https://akidwa.ie/our-work/

Founded in the late 1990s/early 2000s, AkiDwA advocates for migrant women in Ireland, designing initiatives that help them gain access to resources and informing research and policy development nationwide.

Alliance for Choice

http://www.alliance4choice.com/

Since 1996, Alliance for Choice has advocated and campaigned for women's access to sexual and reproductive health services in Ireland as well as for those women seeking abortions in Britain. It focuses on making free, safe, legal, and local abortion available to all.

Archiving the 8th

https://archivingthe8th.ucd.ie

Archiving the 8th is a collection of academics, activists, and archivists who organized after the abortion referendum of 2018 with the goal of documenting abortion activism from the Eighth Amendment through the Repeal campaign. Housed digitally at University College Dublin, it provides resources on where people can donate documents and ephemera related to abortion.

CervicalCheck

https://www.cervicalcheck.ie/

CervicalCheck is the National Cervical Screening Programme organized by the Health Services Executive (HSE), Ireland. Its goal is to reduce the number of Irish people with cervical cancer through a government-sponsored screening program. It offers a free cervical screening test to all people with a cervix between the ages of 25 and 65.

Community Midwives Association

http://communitymidwives.ie/

The Community Midwives Association of Ireland advocates for midwife-led home birth. It also provides home birth services for women through Self-Employed Community Midwives via the Health Service Executive (HSE).

Dublin Well Woman Centre

https://wellwomancentre.ie

Founded in 1978, when both abortion and contraception were not permitted in Ireland, the Dublin Well Woman Centre, which currently has three locations, provides healthcare for all women, with a focus on sexual health.

Doctors for Choice Ireland

https://doctorsforchoiceireland.com

The motto of Doctors for Choice Ireland is "pro-woman, pro-child, pro-choice." It is a coalition of medical professionals who advocate for safe healthcare, including abortion, for all women. Many members of Doctors for Choice campaigned for the Repeal of the Eighth Amendment in 2018.

Elephant Collective

https://www.facebook.com/The-Elephant-Collective-166266716 3990925/

The Elephant Collective, created in 2014, is a group of birth activists, midwives, and artists who work to raise awareness about, and improvements to, Ireland's maternal health system. It particularly has called attention to maternal deaths in Ireland and has successfully campaigned for automatic state inquests following all maternal deaths.

Everyday Stories

https://www.facebook.com/EverydayStoriesIrl/

Everyday Stories began as an affiliate group of the Together for Yes campaign and was a member of the Coalition to Repeal the

Eighth. Through story-telling and illustration, it attempts to highlight the damaging effects of the Eighth Amendment.

Global Advisory Committee on Vaccine Safety (GACVS)

https://www.who.int/groups/global-advisory-committee-on-vacc ine-safety/

The GACVS is a World Health Organization advisory committee, providing scientific, impartial advice on vaccines and vaccine safety globally.

Heath Information and Quality Authority (HIQA)

https://www.hiqa.ie

The HIQA is an independent authority in Ireland that reports to the Minister for Health. Its goal is to improve high-quality and safe health and social services for all Irish people.

Health Service Executive (HSE)

https://www.hse.ie/eng/

The HSE runs all of the public health services in Ireland. Led by the Minister for Health, the HSE provides health and personal social care services to the general public through Divisions, hospital groups, and community health organizations.

In Her Shoes—Women of the Eighth

https://www.facebook.com/InHerIrishShoes

In Her Shoes—Women of the Eighth was launched to support Repeal by sharing the anonymous stories of women and girls who were impacted by the Eighth Amendment and forced to travel or seek illegal abortion pills. Following repeal of the Eighth Amendment, *In Her Shoes* continues to advocate for reproductive autonomy for women in Ireland and around the world.

In Our Shoes—Covid Pregnancy

https://www.facebook.com/inourshoescovidpregnancy/

Via Facebook and Twitter, *In Our Shoes—Covid Pregnancy* spreads awareness about the pregnancy-related restrictions brought by the COVID-19 pandemic.

International Federation of Gynaecology and Obstetrics (FIGO)
https://www.figo.org/
The FIGO brings together obstetrician and gynecologist professional societies from around the world to improve women's
health and rights and to reduce disparities in healthcare.

Irish Family Planning Association (IFPA)
https://www.ifpa.ie/
The IFPA is Ireland's leading sexual and reproductive health services
provider, offering comprehensive care such as contraception,
pregnancy counseling, abortion care, sexually transmitted infection screening, cervical screening, menopause care, vasectomy,
and more. For over fifty years, the IFPA has supported the highest standard of sexual and reproductive health and rights.

Justice for Magdalene Research
http://jfmresearch.com/
Justice for Magdalene (2003–2013) was a not-for-profit, volunteer-
run survivor advocacy group that achieved a compensation
redress scheme for all Magdalene survivors and an official apology from the Irish State. Today, Justice for Magdalene Research
provides support to survivors and their families, as well as education on human rights abuse through research on the Magdalene
Laundries and similar institutions.

Midwives Association of Ireland (MAI)
http://midwivesireland.ie/
The MAI is a professional membership association that advocates for
and empowers midwives to support women through evidence-
based care.

Midwives for Choice
https://www.facebook.com/midwives4choice/
Midwives for Choice worked to repeal the Eighth Amendment
and to advocate for improved reproductive and birth rights
for women.

Migrants and Ethnic-minorities for Reproductive Justice (MERJ)

https://merjireland.org

Founded in 2017 by migrant women of color, MERJ created a platform for the often-hidden voices of migrant and ethnic minority women, nonbinary, and trans people in Ireland and continues to transform feminist discourse in Ireland.

Mother and Baby Homes Commission

https://www.gov.ie/en/collection/mbhcoi/

The Commission of Investigation into Mother and Baby Homes (2015–2021) provided a report of what happened to vulnerable women and children in Mother and Baby Homes from 1922 to 1998.

National Traveller Women's Forum (NTWF)

https://www.ntwf.net/

The NTWF is an alliance of Traveller women and organizations working collectively to challenge racism and sexism experienced by Traveller women and promote Traveller women's human rights and equality.

National Women and Infants Health Programme

https://www.hse.ie/eng/about/who/acute-hospitals-division/woman-infants/

Since 2017, the National Women and Infants Health Programme has led the management, organization, and delivery of maternity, gynecology, and neonatal services in Ireland.

National Women's Council of Ireland (NWC)

https://www.nwci.ie/

Since 1973, the NWC has served as a movement-building membership organization for women and women's groups in Ireland to protect and advance women's and girls' rights domestically and internationally.

Pavee Point Traveller and Roma Centre

https://www.paveepoint.ie/

Pavee Point is an Irish nongovernmental organization employing a collective community development approach to address Traveller and Roma issues and promote Traveller and Roma rights at local, regional, national, and international levels.

Pregnancy Justice

www.pregnancyjustice.org

Formerly known as National Advocates for Pregnant Women, Pregnancy Justice is a US-based nonprofit advocacy organization focused on the human and civil rights, health and welfare of all people, with a focus on pregnant and parenting women.

Rally for Choice Ireland

https://www.facebook.com/rallyforchoice

Rally for Choice Ireland fosters public debate and concerted efforts on the issue of abortion, comprehensive sex education in schools, contraceptive rights, regulation of counseling services to prohibit rogue crisis pregnancy agencies, and ending discrimination of pregnant women in the workplace.

Rape Crisis Network Ireland (RCNI)

https://www.rcni.ie/

The RCNI is "a specialist information and resource centre on rape and all forms of sexual violence." Through national data and research, representation and partnerships, best-practice rape crisis centers, prevention of social violence, and justice, the RCNI aims to eradicate all forms of violence against women and sexual violence.

ROSA Socialist Feminist Movement

https://rosaireland.nationbuilder.com/

ROSA Socialist Feminist Movement is an Irish pro-choice activist group challenging gender and racial oppression, exploitation, inequality and capitalism.

Sexual Health and Crisis Pregnancy Programme (SHCPP)

https://www.hse.ie/eng/about/who/healthwellbeing/our-prior
ity-programmes/sexual-health/

The SHCPP is a national program responsible for implementing
Ireland's National Sexual Health Strategy to improve sexual
health and well-being and to reduce negative sexual health
outcomes.

SisterSong

https://www.sistersong.net/

SisterSong is the national women of color reproductive justice collective in the United States. By strengthening and amplifying the
voices of Indigenous women and women of color, SisterSong
aims to eradicate reproductive oppression, secure human rights,
and achieve reproductive justice.

Survivors of Symphysiotomy

https://www.facebook.com/SoS-Survivors-of-Symphysiotomy-
173631906029192/

Survivors of Symphysiotomy is an activist and advocacy group made
up of survivors of the procedure and their family members. It
was founded in 2001 to push for "truth and justice" in the government's response to the history of symphysiotomy.

Together for Yes

https://www.togetherforyes.ie

Together for Yes is the nationwide umbrella organization that
campaigned to remove the Eighth Amendment from the Irish
Constitution. Comprised of more than seventy groups across
Ireland, it was instrumental in helping to pass the abortion referendum in May 2018.

TranScribe Health Coalition

https://www.transcribehealthcare.org

TranScribe Health Coalition is a group that advocates for trans
equality in healthcare based on informed consent. It provides a

platform for trans people to tell their healthcare stories anonymously and thus safely.

United Nations Population Fund (UNFPA)

https://www.unfpa.org

The UNFPA is the unit of the United Nations that focuses on sexual and reproductive health. Its mission is "to deliver a world where every pregnancy is wanted, every childbirth is safe and every young person's potential is fulfilled."

Women Help Women

https://womenhelp.org

Women Help Women is a nonprofit organization that supports self-induced medical abortion and increased access to abortion pills. Its focus is on "putting abortion pills directly into the hands of those that need them."

Women on Waves

https://www.womenonwaves.org/

Founded by Dr. Rebecca Gomperts in 1999, Women on Waves provides abortion services on ships and through robots and drones, as well as offering workshops and developing art projects.

Women on Web

https://www.womenonweb.org

Founded by Dr. Rebecca Gomperts in 2005, Women on Web is a Canadian nonprofit organization that provides telemedicine access to contraception, as well as mifepristone and misoprostol in countries without safe termination of pregnancy care.

Women's Collective Ireland

https://womenscollective.ie

Created in 2002 and funded by the Irish government's Department of Children, Equality, Disability, Integration, and Youth, Women's Collective Ireland works to improve the lives of women facing marginalization and inequality, particularly through community development.

World Health Organization (WHO)

https://www.who.int

The WHO is an international organization focused on improving human health globally. According to its website, it "leads and champions global efforts to give everyone, everywhere an equal chance to live a healthy life."

INDEX

For the benefit of digital users, indexed terms that span two pages (e.g., 52–53) may, on occasion, appear on only one of those pages.

ABA (An Bord Altranais), 165
A. B. and C. v. Ireland, 82–83
abortion. *See also* Eighth Amendment;
    Health (Regulation of Pregnancy) Act,
    2018; Repeal campaign
    A. B. and C. v. Ireland on, 82–83
    Archiving the 8th on, 102
    Catholic Church and, 81
    Citizen's Assembly on the Eighth
        Amendment and, 58
    "conscientious objection" clause and, 100
    contraception activism linked to, 46–
        48, 71
    COVID-19 pandemic and access to,
        76, 100–1
    criminal, 78–79
    fatal fetal abnormalities and, 95–96
    Halappanavar's death and, 83–84
    In Her Shoes campaign on, 47–48, 76–77,
        79–80, 87–89
    intersectionality and access to, 76
    legalizing, 17
    migrant women access to, 97
    Offences Against the Person Act on,
        77–78, 81
    online trolls and, 90–92
    Protection of Life During Pregnancy Act
        on, 83–84
    reproductive justice and, 79
    Roe v. Wade and, 81
    "shame-industrial complex" and, 78–79
    social media advocacy on, 88–90
    telemedicine, 187
    Thirteenth and Fourteenth Amendments
        on, 81–82
    travel and, 78–82, 95
    truth-telling on, 84–92
    voices in activism for, 92–98
    "X" case on, 81–82
abortion pills, 95, 101
Abortion Rights Campaign, 85
"abortion trail" to UK, 78–79
abstinence, 62–63
Aid Access, 187–88
AIMS (Association for Improvements in the
    Maternity Services), 183
AITHS (All Ireland Traveller Health
    Study), 147
AkiDwA, 53
All Ireland Traveller Health Study
    (AITHS), 147
Allison, Jill, 114–15

An Bord Altranais (ABA), 165
archival research, 6–7
Archiving the 8th, 102
Artists' Campaign to Repeal the Eighth
    Amendment, 86
arts activism, for Repeal campaign, 86–87
Assisted Care pathway, for pregnancy, 108–9
Association for Improvements in the
    Maternity Services (AIMS), 183
asylum-seeking women, maternity care
    for, 145–48
Attic Press, 132–33
Aznar, Hugo, 40, 41–42

Baby-Friendly Hospital Initiative
    (BFHI), 148
Bacik, Ivana, 188–89
Bakhru, Tanya Saroj, 10–11
Barry, Arthur, 170–71
Bassel, Hala, 14
Behan, Mathilda, 177
Bender, Abby, 129, 148–49
Bessborough Mother and Baby Home,
    129, 148–50
BFHI (Baby-Friendly Hospital
    Initiative), 148
birth control. *See* contraception
birth control pill, 50, 55, 56, 59, 61, 64, 66–
    68. *See also* contraception
Birth Project Group, 141–42
Birth Stories podcast, 150
Blood Transfusion Services Board
    (BTSB), 25
bodily autonomy
    Catholic Church impact on, 77
    contraception and, 46–48
    human rights and, 184–85
    obstetric violence and, 161, 174–75
    pregnancy and, 110
    symphysiotomies and, 174–75
Boylan, Peter, 94, 103–4, 188–89
Bracken, Claire, 3–4, 89–90
breastfeeding, 148–49
Breastival, 148
Brennan, Laura, 40
Brounéus, Karen, 15

BTSB (Blood Transfusion Services
    Board), 25
"bulk buying" contraception, 52

Cadden, Mamie, 78
Campaign Against Church Ownership of
    Women's Healthcare, 103–4
Canada, Truth and Reconciliation
    Commission, 179–81
capitalism, maternity care and, 141–42
Carlow for Choice, 6
Carroll, Michaela, 80
Castillo-Martin, Marcia, 40, 41–42
Catholic Church
    abortion and, 81
    bodily autonomy and, 77
    cesarean sections and, 170
    contraception and, 50–51, 60–61, 64
    hospital management by, 157–58
    In Our Shoes—Covid Pregnancy campaign
        on, 119
    Mother-and-Child scheme of, 158
    National Maternity Hospital ownership
        of, 103–4
    sexuality regulated by, 60
    symphysiotomies and, 170–72
    women's health and, 13
Central Midwives Board, 166
cervical cancer
    ethical communication on screening
        for, 43
    from HPV, 20, 22–23
    Ireland statistics on, 22–23
    prevention, 16
    public awareness of, 35
    reproductive justice and prevention
        of, 26–27
    Traveller women resisting screening
        for, 26–27
    women's health stigmatization and, 28–
        29, 37–38
Cervical Cancer Vaccine–Is It Safe?, 36–37
CervicalCheck, 1, 20
    legal cases filed against, 30–31
    MERJ on, 29–30, 45
    redress and, 34–35

Scally Report on failings of, 20–21, 23,
28–29, 30, 42
scandal with, 16, 22–23, 28–32
successes of, 31
truth-telling and, 32–36
unethical communication and, 21–22
Varadkar apologizing for failures
of, 31–32
women-first approach for, 30
women's health improvements after
scandal of, 35–36
CervicalCheck Tribunal, 44–45
cesarean sections
Catholic Church and, 170
rates of, 130, 142–43
childbirth. *See also* maternity care; obstetric
violence
breastfeeding and, 148–49
Catholic Church on cesarean, 170
cesarean section, 130, 142–43, 170
COVID-19 pandemic restrictions for,
119, 120
disruptive factors to, 120–21
Elephant Collective and, 136–37, 138–39
at home, 107, 130–31
in hospital, 106–7, 130–31
improving, 150–52
In Our Shoes—Covid Pregnancy campaign
on contemporary, 139–41
MAMMI study on, 142–44
maternal death and, 18, 135–39
miscarriage and, 124–25, 145–47
natural compared to medicalized, 144–
45, 150
reproductive justice and, 131–35
SisterSong and, 133–34
Traveller and asylum-seeking women
and, 145–48
truth-telling on, 135–39
well-being association with, 142–43
World Patient Safety Day and, 119–20
Children and Family Relationships Act,
2015, 114–15
Citizen's Assembly on the Eighth
Amendment, 58, 84
Clark, Maureen Harding, 183

Coalition for Improving Maternity Services
and Childbirth Connection, 142–43
Coalition to Repeal the Eighth
Amendment, 85
coercion, contraception and, 71
colonialism
in Ireland and handywomen, 12–13
obstetric violence and, 161–62
symphysiotomies and, 161–62
Committee on Evil Literature, 61
Conaghan, Joanne, 92–93, 175
condoms, 50, 55, 66–68. *See also*
contraception
*Confidential Maternal Death Enquiry in
Ireland*, 145–46
Connolly, Linda, 64–65
Conroy, Róisín, 132–33
"conscientious objection" clause, 100
Considine, Maureen, 149–50
contraception
abortion activism linked to, 46–48, 71
access to, 16–17
barriers to effective use of, 49–50
bodily autonomy and, 46–48
"bulk buying," 52
Catholic Church and, 50–51, 60–61, 64
Citizen's Assembly on the Eighth
Amendment and, 58
coercion and, 71
Committee on Evil Literature on, 61
cost of, 52, 55–57, 68
crisis pregnancies from lack of, 48–49
decriminalization of, 61
Direct Provision and access to, 54
Eighth Amendment and, 61–62
failure rates of, 49–50, 67–68
feminist activism and, 64–65
free, 46, 73
history and truth-telling on, 57–66
hormonal, 59
ignorance on, 49–51, 62–64, 72
In Her Shoes campaign on, 47–48, 56,
63, 67–68
legal prohibitions on, 59–60, 64
long-acting reversible, 47, 56, 59, 68–71
media scaremongering on, 58–59

contraception (*cont.*)
  mifepristone as, 190
  migrant women and, 51–54
  popular methods of, 56–57
  public campaigns on, 57
  rates of use, 46
  reproductive justice and, 48–57, 63, 71
  shared responsibility of, 49
  social media advocacy on, 66
  sterilization and, 61–62
  Traveller women and, 51–52, 54–55
  truth-telling on, 72
  types of, 66–71
  in US, 61
  women's liberation linked to, 64
  Working Group on Access to, 46, 50–51,
    57–58, 72–73
Contraception Action Program (CAP), 64
"contraception scare," 58–59
Contract Against Cancer, 39
Coombe Maternity Hospital, 171
Cooney, Patrick, 61
Cork Mother Jones Committee, 129
Cork Survivors and Supporters Alliance
  (CSSA), 129, 149–50
Coroners (Amendment) Act 2019, 1, 18,
  130–31, 136–37, 138
COVID-19 pandemic, 17. See also *In Our
  Shoes—Covid Pregnancy* campaign
  abortion access during, 76, 100–1
  childbirth restrictions from, 119, 120
  domestic violence during, 117
  maternity care during, 104–5, 116–17,
    119, 120, 127–28
  mental health of women during, 116–17,
    118–19, 122–23, 126
  vaccination rates for, 121
  women's health and, 17–18, 116–17, 126–27
Creating a Better Future Together, 107–8
criminal abortions, 78–79
crisis pregnancies
  contraception lacking in, 48–49
  stealthing causing, 68
  travel and, 80
Crosby, Alison, 15
CSSA (Cork Survivors and Supporters
  Alliance), 129, 149–50

Cullen, Pauline, 127–28
Cutter, Noelle, 114

DAHR (donor-assisted human
  reproduction), 114–15
Daly, Clare, 136–37
Delay, Cara, 3–4, 81, 89–90
Denmark, 37
Diaz-Tello, Farah, 160
Direct Provision
  contraception access in, 54
  maternity care and, 113–14
  as "shame-industrial complex" heir, 5
Dobbs v. Jackson Women's Health, 188–89
document analysis, 6–7
domestic violence, 117
Domiciliary In and Out (DOMINO)
  care, 106–7
Donnelly, Stephen, 46
donor-assisted human reproduction
  (DAHR), 114–15
"Don't Be Swayed by Rumors" video, 41
door-to-door canvassing, 85–86
Drugs Payment Scheme, 114

Edwards, Nadine, 126–27, 141–42
Eighth Amendment. See also Repeal
  campaign
  adoption of, 81
  Archiving the 8th on, 102
  Citizen's Assembly on, 58, 84
  contraception and, 61–62
  legacy of, 184
  legal challenges to, 81–84
  maternity care and, 110, 115
  referendum on, 84
  repeal of, 1
  "X" case on, 81–82
Elephant Collective, 18, 136–37, 138–
  39, 184
empowerment, through truth-telling, 45
Enright, Máiréad, 176–77, 178
Equal Status Act, 2002, 147
ethical communication
  beneficence from, 40
  on cervical cancer screening, 43
  HPV Vaccination Alliance and, 45

for reproductive justice, 21–22
truth-telling and, 45
for women-first approach, 44
European Convention on Human
    Rights, 10–11·

Facebook, 7, 90, 91, 117–18, 177. See also *In
    Her Shoes* campaign
fatal fetal abnormalities, 95–96
feminist activism. See also *In Her Shoes*
    campaign; *In Our Shoes—Covid
    Pregnancy* campaign
    arts and, 86–87
    contraception and, 64–65
    door-to-door canvassing and, 85–86
    historical achievements of, 93
    intersectionality and, 132–33, 134–35
    Repeal campaign building on history
        of, 92–93
    research methods in, 8–9
    story-telling-as-strategy in, 75–76,
        85, 94–95
FIGO (International Federation of
    Gynaecology and Obstetrics), 119–20
Fischer, Clara, 3–4, 12–13, 29, 32–33,
    51, 78–79
Fitzpatrick, Laura, 7
forced hysterectomies
    government apology for, 167–68
    midwives and, 165–66
    misogyny and, 166–67
    Neary performing, 153–54, 158–59, 163–
        68, 175–76
    patient stories of, 163–64
    process of, 163
    "shame-industrial complex" and, 154–55
    truth-telling on, 175–76
Fourteenth Amendment, 81–82

Gallen, James, 4, 15
Gernon, Corah, 150
Gomperts, Rebecca, 187–88, 190
Greene, Anne-Marie, 7, 136–37
Greene, Jo, 187
The Guardian, 83–84

Halappanavar, Savita, 10–12, 83–84

handywomen, colonialism in Ireland
    and, 12–13
Hanlon, Steph, 6
Harris, Simon, 31–32
Harte, Michelle, 82–83
Haughey, Caoimhe, 138
Health (Regulation of Pregnancy) Act,
    2018, 17
    government review of, 101–2
    limitations of, 99
    MERJ on, 100
Healthcare Pricing Office, 145–46
Health Service Executive (HSE), 23, 53,
    107, 116
Healthy Ireland, 112–13
Healthy People guidelines, US, 37
hepatitis C scandal, 25
Higgins, Maeve, 1, 190
Higgins, Michael D., 148
Higgins, Sabina, 148
HIQA (Irish Health Information and
    Quality Authority), 107–9, 111–12
Hogan, Caelainn, 2–3, 78–79, 154–55
homebirths, 107, 130–31
hormonal contraception, 59
"hormonophobia," 59
hospital birth, 106–7, 130–31
HPV. *See* human papillomavirus
HPV Vaccination Alliance, 28, 39, 41–42, 45
HPV vaccination misinformation campaign,
    16, 20–21
    central lesson of, 41–42
    cervical cancer stigmatization and, 37–38
    Cervical Cancer Vaccine–Is It Safe?
        and, 36–37
    countering, 26–27, 39–40
    emotional manipulation of parents
        in, 38–39
    impact of, 24–25
    international spread of, 37
    mission of, 24
    truth-telling against, 41–42
    unethical communication and, 21–22
    vaccine hesitancy and, 24
#HPVVAXFACTS campaign, 39
HSE (Health Service Executive), 23, 53,
    107, 116

Humanae Vitae, 61, 81
Human Life Is Sacred, 81
human papillomavirus (HPV). *See also* HPV
   vaccination misinformation campaign
   cervical cancer from, 20, 22–23
   cervical cancer stigmatization and, 37–38
   incidence of, 24
human rights
   bodily autonomy and, 184–85
   European Convention on, 10–11
   in Ireland, 10–13
   obstetric violence and, 159
   reproductive justice and, 9–13, 25
   Universal Declaration on, 142–43
   women's rights as, 9
Hyesun Hwang, 89
Hynan, Martina, 136–37
hysterectomies. *See* forced hysterectomies

ICPD (International Conference on
   Population and Development), 9
identity, pregnancy, power and, 17–18
IFPA (Irish Family Planning Association),
   10–11, 54, 101
I.M.E.L.D.A., 87
India Times, 83
infertility, 114
Inglis, Tom, 50–51
In Her Shoes campaign, 1–2, 17–18
   on abortion, 47–48, 76–77, 79–80, 87–89
   Archiving the 8th on, 102
   on contraception, 56, 63, 67–68
   Repeal Shield tool for, 90–91, 186
   spam accounts against, 90
   in IVF (vitro fertilization), 114
In Our Shoes—Covid Pregnancy campaign,
   104–5, 119–26, 184
   analyzing posts from, 121
   Catholic Church and, 119
   on companion restrictions, 121–22,
      124, 125–26
   on contemporary childbirth, 139–41
   creation and purpose of, 117–18
   disruptions shared in, 121–22
   on guilt, 123
   on miscarriage, 124–25
   on NICU and isolation, 122–23

   revelations of, 128
   on trauma, 123–24
   truth-telling with, 117–19
Instagram, 117–18
International Conference on Population and
   Development (ICPD), 9
International Federation of Gynaecology
   and Obstetrics (FIGO), 119–20
intersectionality, 4–5
   abortion access and, 76
   feminist activism and, 132–33, 134–35
   maternity care and, 115–16
   obstetric violence and, 153
   social media advocacy and, 21–22
interviews, 6–9
intimate partner violence, 117
intrauterine devices (IUDs), 66–67, 69, 70.
   See also contraception
in vitro fertilization (IVF), 114
Ireland. *See also specific topics*
   Catholic Church and women's
      health in, 13
   cervical cancer statistics in, 22–23
   handywomen and colonialism in, 12–13
   remedies for scandals in, 33
   reproductive justice and human rights
      in, 10–13
   social media advocacy in, 16
   transitional justice in, 13–14
   women's health activism in US and model
      of, 188–90
Irish Countrywoman's Association, 64–65
Irish Examiner, 188–89
Irish Family Planning Association (IFPA),
   10–11, 54, 101
Irish Health Information and Quality
   Authority (HIQA), 107–9, 111–12
Irish Housewives' Association, 64–65
Irish Medical Journal, 55
The Irish Times, 183
Irish Women's Liberation Movement
   (IWLM), 64, 65
Irish Women United (IWU), 64, 132–33
IUDs (intrauterine devices), 66–67, 69, 70.
   See also contraception
IWLM (Irish Women's Liberation
   Movement), 64, 65

IWU (Irish Women United), 64

Japan, 37
Jardine, Robert, 169–70
Jones, Mary Harris ("Mother Jones"), 129
Justice for Magdalens, 4

Kee-Ok Kim, 89
Keller, Jessalynn, 15
Kelly, Laura, 64, 93
Kennedy, Patricia, 146–47
Keown, Bridget, 6
Kirkham, Mavis, 141–42

Lamaze International, 142–43
LARC (long-acting reversible
    contraception), 47, 56, 59, 68–71
Lawyers for Choice, 134
Leiva, Gonzalo, 120
Lentín, Ronit, 51–52
LGBTQ people
    DAHR for, 114–15
    same-sex marriage and, 1, 85–86
    trans issues and, 5, 97–98, 186–87
    women's health activism and, 184–85
Londras, Fiona de, 5
long-acting reversible contraception
    (LARC), 47, 56, 59, 68–71
Loughnane, Cliona, 43
Loughrey, Mark, 168
Luibhéid, Eithne, 113–14
Luna, Zakiya, 25, 134
Lykes, M. Brinton, 15
Lynch, Krysia, 145–46

MacCraith, Brian, 30, 42
Magdalene laundries, 1, 2–3, 4, 13–14, 179
Maher, Alice, 86
Mahon, Evelyn, 114
Mahony, Rhona, 94
Malta, 189–90
MAMMI (Maternal Health and Maternal
    Morbidity in Ireland) study, 142–44
Mander, Rosemary, 126–27, 141–
    42, 166–67
marriage
    obstetric violence and, 153

pregnancy and, 63
same-sex, 1, 85–86
Martin, Emily, 157
Maser mural, 86, 87
maternal death, 18, 135–39, 145–46
Maternal Health and Maternal Morbidity in
    Ireland (MAMMI) study, 142–44
Maternity and Infant Care Scheme, 106–7
maternity care. See also In Our Shoes—Covid
    Pregnancy campaign; obstetric violence
    for asylum-seeking women, 145–48
    breastfeeding and, 148–49
    capitalism and, 141–42
    Catholic Church's Mother-and-Child
        scheme and, 158
    COVID-19 pandemic restrictions for,
        104–5, 116–17, 119, 120, 127–28
    crisis in, 139–45
    DAHR and, 114–15
    Direct Provision and, 113–14
    DOMINO care and, 106–7
    Eighth Amendment and, 110, 115
    FIGO's framework for, 119–20
    historical development of, 105–6, 141
    in hospital, 106–7
    improving, 150–52
    infertility and, 114
    integrated, 110–11
    intersectionality and, 115–16
    location-based disparities in, 113–14
    MAMMI study on, 142–44
    MERJ on, 139
    miscarriage and, 124–25, 145–47
    National Strategy for, 107–9, 110–12, 116
    pathways for, 108–9
    reproductive justice and, 112–17
    for Traveller women, 113–14, 145–48
    truth-telling and, 117–19
    ultrasound services for, 111–12
    woman-centered, 105–12, 143–44
    World Patient Safety Day and, 119–20
McAuliffe, Mary, 42
McAvoy, Sandra, 61
McCann, Rita, 153–54
McCarthy, Joan, 168
McCole, Brigid, 25
McEnroy, Monica, 13

McEvoy, Karen, 135–36, 138
McGaughey, Fiona, 147–48
McNaull, G., 138
McQuade, Shirley, 48–49
media, "contraception scare" in, 58–59
Mendes, Kaitlynn, 15
mental health of women, during COVID-19
    pandemic, 116–17, 118–19, 122–
    23, 126
MERJ. *See* Migrants and Ethnic-minorities
    for Reproductive Justice
midwives, forced hysterectomies
    and, 165–66
Midwives Association of Ireland, 120–
    21, 127–28
mifepristone, as contraception, 190
Migrants and Ethnic-minorities for
    Reproductive Justice (MERJ)
    on CervicalCheck, 29–30, 45
    on Health (Regulation of Pregnancy) Act,
        2018, 100
    on maternal death of migrant
        women, 137
    on maternity care, 139
    on miscarriage, 146–47
    mission of, 5
    on Repeal campaign exclusion, 97, 98
migrant women. *See also* Traveller women
    abortion access and, 97
    AkiDwA study on, 53
    contraception and, 51–54
    maternal death of, 137, 145–46
    maternity care for, 145–48
    Repeal campaign and, 97, 98
    reproductive justice challenges of, 11–12
miscarriage, 124–25, 145–47
Mishler, Katie, 85, 96–97
misinformation. *See* HPV vaccination
    misinformation campaign
misogyny
    forced hysterectomies and, 166–67
    institutionalized, 42
    in women's health, 3–4
Missing and Murdered Indigenous Women
    and Girls (MMIWG), Canada, 179–80
Molloy, Catriona, 176
Morrissey, Jacqueline, 176–77

Mother and Baby Homes, 1, 2–3, 4, 13–14,
    130, 139, 148–50, 179
Mother-and-Child scheme, 1950s, 158
"Mother Jones" (Mary Harris Jones), 129
Mother Jones magazine, 129
Murphy, Mary, 127–28
Murphy, Sharon, 168
Murphy-Lawless, Jo, 10–11, 126–27, 136–
    37, 138–39, 141–42, 146–47, 166–67

National Institute for Health and Care
    Excellence (NICE), 142–43
National Maternity Hospital, , 103–4, 170
National Maternity Strategy, 107–9, 110–
    12, 116
*National Standards for Safer Better Maternity
    Services*, 107–8
National Women's Council, 43, 85, 181–82
Neary, Michael, 153–54, 158–59, 163–
    68, 175–76
neonatal intensive care unit
    (NICU), 122–23
neonatal mortality rate, 145–46
New York Times, 1
Ní Aoláin, Fionnuala, 180–81
NICE (National Institute for Health and
    Care Excellence), 142–43
NICU (neonatal intensive care
    unit), 122–23
nonbinary people, 5

obstetric violence, 18–19. *See also* forced
    hysterectomies; symphysiotomies
    bodily autonomy and, 161, 174–75
    colonialism and, 161–62
    definition of, 160
    government response to, 179
    historical development of, 156–
        57, 161–62
    human rights and, 159
    intersectionality and, 153
    long-term effects of, 181–82
    marriage and, 153
    post-traumatic stress disorder from, 172
    pubiotomies and, 153–54, 172
    reproductive justice and, 154–62
    "shame-industrial complex" and, 154–55

transitional justice and, 179
truth-telling on, 175–81
O'Connor, Marie, 172
O'Connor, Orla, 181–82
O'Connor, Sheila, 158–59, 169
O'Donnell, Katherine, 2–3, 179
OECD (Organisation for Economic Co-operation and Development), 130
Offences Against the Person Act, 1861, UK, 77–78, 81
O'Hara, Lorna, 86
Olza, Ibone, 120
Onanuga, Bimbo, 11–12
online trolls, 90–92, 186
Organisation for Economic Co-operation and Development (OECD), 130
O'Rourke, Maeve, 2–3, 179
O'Rourke, Sinéad, 183
O'Shaughnessy, Aideen, 95
O'Shea, Brendan, 31
Our Lady of Lourdes Hospital, 18–19, 158–59, 163–68, 175–76

parents, HPV vaccination misinformation campaign manipulation of, 38–39
participant observation, 6–7
Patient Safety Bill proposal, 2019, 44–45
patriarchy, in women's health, 44
perinatal mortality rate (PMR), 145–46
Perinatal Statistics Report, 145–46
Personal Public Service (PPS), 45
Phelan, Vicky, 23, 27–28, 30, 40, 42–43
Picking up the Threads, 7, 136–37
PMR (perinatal mortality rate), 145–46
Poland, 92
politics of shame, 29, 51
Positive Action, 25
post-traumatic stress disorder, from obstetric violence, 172
power, pregnancy, identity and, 17–18
PPS (Personal Public Service), 45
pregnancy. See also childbirth; crisis pregnancies; In Our Shoes—Covid Pregnancy campaign; maternity care; obstetric violence
bodily autonomy and, 110
during COVID-19 pandemic, 104–5

DAHR for, 114–15
DOMINO care and, 106–7
hospital admission and, 106–7
identity, power and, 17–18
infertility and, 114
marriage and, 63
miscarriage and, 124–25
pathways for, 108–9
Protection of Life During Pregnancy Act and, 83–84
rates, 130
reproductive justice and, 112–17
SEP and, 112–13
surrogacy and, 114–15
truth-telling and, 117–19
Price, Kimala, 9–10
Protection of Life During Pregnancy Act, 2013, 83–84
pubiotomies, 153–54, 172
purposive sampling, 7–8

Ralph, David, 83
RCOG (Royal College of Obstetricians and Gynecologists), 30–31
Rebel Women magazine, 132–33
redress, truth-telling for, 34–35
Reid, Bernadette, 54–55, 73, 147–48
religious health services, 44
Religious Sisters of Charity, 103–4
Repeal campaign, 17. See also Eighth Amendment; Health (Regulation of Pregnancy) Act, 2018
Archiving the 8th on, 102
arts activism for, 86–87
door-to-door canvassing of, 85–86
fatal fetal abnormality stories in, 95–96
feminist activism history and, 92–93
global implications of, 92
groups for, 85
legacy of, 135, 184
methods of, 74–75, 87, 94
migrant women and, 97, 98
mobilization of, 74–75
online trolls and, 90–92
social media advocacy for, 88–90
success of, 74–76, 92–93
trans people and, 97–98

Repeal campaign (*cont.*)
  truth-telling in, 84–85
  voices in, 92–98
Repeal Shield tool, 90–91, 186
reproductive justice
  abortion and, 79
  cervical cancer prevention and, 26–27
  childbirth and, 131–35
  contraception and, 48–57, 63, 71
  definition of, 9
  ethical communication for, 21–22
  evolution of, 131–33
  human rights and, 9–13, 25
  in Ireland, 10–13
  Lawyers for Choice on, 134
  migrant women challenges in, 11–12
  movement for, 9
  National Maternity Strategy and, 116
  obstetric violence and, 154–62
  pregnancy, maternity care and, 112–17
  redress and, 34–35
  social justice issues connected to, 9–10
  Traveller women and, 11–12
  truth-telling and, 14, 15, 27–28, 184
  violence and, 9–10
  women's health activism and, 11
research methods, 6–9
Ringrose, Jessica, 15
Roe v. Wade, 81, 188–89, 190
Rolston, Bill, 180–81
Ross, Loretta, 89
Rosser, Emily, 34–35
Royal College of Obstetricians and
    Gynecologists (RCOG), 30–31
Russell, Noirin, 30–31
Rwanda, 15

Sadler, Michelle, 120, 159–60
same-sex marriage, 1, 85–86
San Marino, 189–90
Scally Report, 20–21, 23, 28–29, 30, 42
Scranton, P., 138
Sebesta, Amanda, 21–22
SEP (socioeconomic position), pregnancy
    and, 112–13
sexuality
  Catholic Church regulating, 60

  marriage and, 63
  moralistic approach to, 42, 44, 110
  politics of shame and, 29, 51
sexually transmitted infections (STIs),
    24, 37–38. *See also* human
    papillomavirus
Shabot, Sarah Cohen, 174–75, 181–82
"shame-industrial complex," 2–4, 5, 78–
    79, 154–55
Sherlock, Leslie, 184
Side, Katherine, 51–52, 89–90, 92–93
Silent Killer, 7
Simms, Kate, 24
Sisters of Mercy, 157–58
SisterSong, 9, 133–34
Sky News, 83
Smith, James M., 2–3, 162, 179
Smyly, W. J., 169–70
Smyth, Ailbhe, 99, 188–89
snowball sampling, 7–8
social media advocacy. See also *In Her
    Shoes* campaign; *In Our Shoes—Covid
    Pregnancy* campaign
  on contraception, 66
  of I.M.E.L.D.A., 87
  intersectionality and, 21–22
  in Ireland, 16
  online trolls and, 90–92, 186
  for Repeal campaign, 88–90
  Repeal Shield tool for, 90–91, 186
  truth-telling and, 15–16, 27–28
  women's health activism and, 4–5, 7
socioeconomic position (SEP), pregnancy
    and, 112–13
solidarity-discord identity paradox, 21–22
Solinger, Rickie, 89
SOS (Survivors of
    Symphysiotomy), 176–78
Spain, Alex, 170–71
Specialized Care pathway, for
    pregnancy, 108–9
Spillane, Alison, 101
Spirit of Mother Jones Award, 129
stealthing, crisis pregnancies from, 68
sterilization, 61–62
STIs (sexually transmitted infections), 24,
    37–38. *See also* human papillomavirus

story-telling-as-strategy, in feminist activism, 75–76, 85, 94–95
Supported Care pathway, for pregnancy, 108–9
surrogacy, pregnancy and, 114–15
Survivors of Symphysiotomy (SOS), 176–78
survivor voices, 4
symphysiotomies, 153–54
  bodily autonomy and, 174–75
  Catholic Church and, 170–72
  colonialism and, 161–62
  historical practice of, 169–70
  incidence of, 172
  patient accounts of, 169, 171–72, 173–74
  post-traumatic stress disorder from, 172
  process of, 169
  secrecy surrounding, 176–77
  "shame-industrial complex" and, 154–55
  truth-telling on, 176–78
  Walsh Report on, 177, 178–79
  women's health activism on, 156, 172–73

targeted regulation of abortion providers (TRAP) laws, US, 187–88
Tariq, Nayyab, 138
Taylor, Julie, 54–55, 73, 147–48
telemedicine abortion, 187
Termination for Medical Reasons (TFMR), 95–96
Thirteenth Amendment, 81–82
Together for Yes movement, 85, 90, 94, 96, 184–85. See also Repeal campaign
TranScribe Health, 186–87
transitional justice
  in Ireland, 13–14
  obstetric violence and, 179
  problems with, 15
  "Troubles" and, 181
  truth-telling and, 13–15
trans people, 5, 97–98, 186–87
TRAP (targeted regulation of abortion providers) laws, US, 187–88
travel, abortion and, 78–82, 95
Traveller women
  breastfeeding barriers and, 148–49
  cervical cancer screenings resisted by, 26–27

contraception and, 51–52, 54–55
Equal Status Act of 2002 and, 147
health disparities of, 147
maternity care for, 113–14, 145–48
reproductive justice and, 11–12
trolls, online, 90–92, 186
"Troubles," transitional justice and, 181
Truth and Reconciliation Commission, Canada, 179–81
truth-telling
  on abortion, 84–92
  CervicalCheck and, 32–36
  on childbirth and maternal death, 135–39
  on contraception, 72
  contraception history and, 57–66
  empowerment through, 45
  ethical communication and, 45
  on forced hysterectomies, 175–76
  on hepatitis C scandal, 25
  against HPV vaccination misinformation campaign, 41–42
  with In Our Shoes—Covid Pregnancy campaign, 117–19
  on obstetric violence, 175–81
  pregnancy, maternity care and, 117–19
  problems with, 15
  for redress, 34–35
  in Repeal campaign, 84–85
  reproductive justice and, 14, 15, 27–28, 184
  social media advocacy and, 15–16, 27–28
  on symphysiotomies, 176–78
  transitional justice and, 13–15
Twitter, 7, 89–90. See also In Her Shoes campaign

UK. See United Kingdom
ultrasound services, 111–12
unethical communication, 21–22
UNHRC (United Nations Human Rights Committee), 83–84
United Kingdom (UK)
  "abortion trail" to, 78–79
  NICE in, 142–43
  Offences Against the Person Act of 1861 and, 77–78, 81

United Nations Human Rights Committee
(UNHRC), 83–84
United States (US)
contraception in, 61
Dobbs v. Jackson Women's Health
in, 188–89
Healthy People guidelines, 37.
Roe v. Wade in, 81, 188–89, 190
TRAP laws in, 187–88
women's health activism in, 19
women's health activism in Ireland as
model for, 188–90
Universal Declaration on Human
Rights, 142–43
US. *See* United States

Vacaflor, Carlos Herrera, 160
vaccine hesitancy, 24
Valera, Éamon De, 171–72
Varadkar, Leo, 31–32
Vardeman, Jennifer, 21–22
violence. *See also* obstetric violence
intimate partner, 117
reproductive justice and, 9–10

Walker, Margaret Urban, 14
Walsh, Lorraine, 35–36
Walsh, Oonagh, 170–71
Walsh Report, 177, 178–79
#WeAreDelivering, 183
Wellcome Trust, 102
Well Woman Centre, 49–50, 67
WHO (World Health Organization), 24–25,
119–21, 130, 150–51, 159
woman-centered maternity care, 105–
12, 143–44
women-first approach
for CervicalCheck, 30
ethical communication for, 44
Women on Waves, 95, 190
Women on Web, 101, 187
women's health

Catholic Church and, 13
cervical cancer stigmatization and, 28–
29, 37–38
CervicalCheck and improvements
for, 35–36
COVID-19 pandemic and, 17–18, 116–
17, 126–27
infertility and, 114
misogyny in, 3–4
patriarchy in, 44
"shame-industrial complex" and, 2–4
survivor voices in, 4
women's health activism. *See also* feminist
activism; *In Her Shoes* campaign; *In
Our Shoes—Covid Pregnancy* campaign
catching fire, 1–2
foundations of, 6
in Ireland as model for US, 188–90
LGBTQ people and, 184–85
against National Maternity
Hospital, 103–4
reproductive justice and, 11
social media advocacy and, 4–5, 7
on symphysiotomies, 156, 172–73
technology changing, 186–87
in United States, 19
Women's Health Taskforce, 151–52
Women's International Information
and Communication Service
Conference, 132–33
women's liberation, contraception
linked to, 64
women's rights, as human rights, 9
Working Group on Access to Contraception,
46, 50–51, 57–58, 72–73
World Health Organization (WHO), 24–25,
119–21, 130, 150–51, 159
World Patient Safety Day, 119–20

"X" case, 81–82

Young, Rachael, 86